The Culture Cure

Intentionally
Create Excellence!

Paula M Tripp

The Culture Cure

TRANSFORMING THE MODERN HEALTHCARE SYSTEM

• • •

Pamela M. Tripp

ISBN: 1533661308
ISBN 13: 9781533661302

Table of Contents

Dedication

• • •

I dedicate this book to my husband and soul mate Danny Paul, and our children Jennifer and Johnathan, for your love and support. To my parents, Royie and Reba, for teaching me about faith in God and living life with purpose. To my Colleagues of CommWell Health, the Eagles through the years that always inspired me to soar to higher altitudes.

Acknowledgments

• • •

There is nothing accomplished in life without the support of many people. A special thanks to the following for helping bring my first book and the ideology of Corporate Transcendence™ to reality.

To God for the desire and inspiration written on my heart. Your faithfulness endureth forever.

To Kary Oberbrunner and Author Academy Elite for guidance and always believing in me.

To the Soaring Eagles and Eagle Mentors who spread their wings to live a life of excellence.

Praise for *The Culture Cure*

• • •

"Pamela has created in this transformational book a way of looking at transforming the healthcare industry through a look at the culture of your organization. An approach is presented which puts both internal and external customers at the forefront. If you are looking for a different way of getting results, try the concepts Pamela is putting forward in transforming your organization! A great read and roadmap."

ANNIE R. NEASMAN, RN, MS PRESIDENT/CEO,
JESSIE TRICE COMMUNITY HEALTH CENTER

"A real life, brass tacks approach to improving relationships, trust, environment and care within healthcare facilities. Hospital and patient experiences will shine bright with the approaches and systems contained in these pages."

MARCUS ENGEL, M.S. AUTHOR OF *THE OTHER END OF THE STETHOSCOPE* AND *I'M HERE: COMPASSIONATE COMMUNICATION IN PATIENT CARE*

"*The Culture Cure* is a must read for any leader who wants to leave a legacy of organizational sustainability and create the best place to work. The discussion around the Corporate

Transcendence™ Transformational Curriculum works well for all business segments including education, nonprofit, manufacturing, small business, government, and healthcare. The power of this book is in hardwiring behavior change by breaking down silos to increase process interdependency; emotionally and intellectually engaging the workforce; and reinforcing accountability. The end result is lasting culture change that ensures a healthy, innovative, thriving organization."

DR. DEBORAH MANZO, CSSBB, ISO, NBCT,
DIRECTOR NC PERFORMANCE EXCELLENCE
PROGRAM, MALCOLM BALDRIGE EXAMINER

"Pamela's book epitomizes Einstein's statement that "Doing the same thing over and over again and expecting different results is insanity." The need for cultural transformation in health care is a critical next step for success, and the book well describes its stifling grip on US health care, as well as a helpful path forward. Throughout the book, the author makes very profound, philosophical, observational statements that truly demonstrate her depth of experience in health care culture. I am walking away from reading this book, empowered and fired up, with a whole new set of valuable tools. I take off my hat to the author!"

TONY AMOFAH, MD, MBA, FACP CHIEF
MEDICAL OFFICER, CHIEF ACADEMIC OFFICER,
COMMUNITY HEALTH OF SOUTH FLORIDA INC.

"Pamela M. Tripp is a graduate of Methodist University's Bachelor of Applied Science program, and an excellent example of what we hope all of our students will become, true leaders who give back to society. She does that well in this new book that addresses the transformation of healthcare through a cultural lens. It asks the question, "How do we transform our traditional culture to meet the demands of healthcare reform?" I know you will find it fascinating and a valuable addition to your library as we continue to address the ever-evolving world of health care reform. Her idea of corporate transcendence is one worthy of consideration."

WARREN G. MCDONALD, PHD PROFESSOR AND CHAIR, HEALTH ADMINISTRATION DEPARTMENT SCHOOL OF HEALTH SCIENCES, METHODIST UNIVERSITY

"When Pam graduated from Johnston Community College and later became a faculty member in Radiography Technology, we all knew she was a leader. Now her study of leadership, also genuinely expressed in her life, has resulted in in a stellar example of thought, process and implementation via the publication of *The Culture Cure: Transforming the Modern Healthcare System.* This is not merely a book about leadership but a work of introspection when, if applied, will assist in transforming leadership into a culture of healing and therefore service. I recommend its reading! But more so, I recommend its application."

DR. DAVID N. JOHNSON, ED.D, PRESIDENT, JOHNSTON COMMUNITY COLLEGE

"This book contributes energy, compassion, and wisdom to the debates about reforming the healthcare system in our country. Rooted in her commitment to exemplify dynamic leadership in her daily work, Tripp's observations and commentary have the force of urgency and authenticity. While some may view her book as idealistic, I have observed her leadership first-hand and I can attest that her vision can be (and should be) reality. Since our health is always a collaborative endeavor, we need more healthcare systems that operate within her vision of a healing culture."

David R. Tillman, PhD, MEd, CPH, Chair & Assistant Professor, Department of Public Health, Campbell University College of Pharmacy & Health Sciences

Introduction

• • •

"Humpty Dumpty sat on a wall; Humpty Dumpty had a great fall. All the kings' horses and all the kings' men could not put Humpty Dumpty back together again."

Healthcare is one of the most controversial social topics across America. Numerous debates and widely diverse opinions exist on the fix needed to support a service industry that mandates excellent patient experience and quality.

The Humpty Dumpty nursery rhyme is a natural analogy to describe the emotions of today's healthcare stakeholders and leaders. Humpty Dumpty sat on a wall; Humpty Dumpty had a great fall. All the kings' horses and all the kings' men could not put Humpty Dumpty back together again.

In this rhyme Humpty Dumpty is depicted as an egg figured character. A dropped egg provides a vivid image of a thin shell body fractured into multiple pieces. A system fractured and where "all the king's horses and all the king's men, couldn't put Humpty together again."

The ongoing debate of healthcare reform and more recent Veterans Administration crisis are prime examples why cultural transformation is needed. Politicians, healthcare leaders and patients agree on one point–that healthcare in America is in need of transformation.

Transformation is never a walk in the park and especially in an industry that has been described by many leadership management experts as one of the most complex industries to lead. There is a public cry for 21st

Century leaders to be front and center and step up to lead the systemic transformation required to obtain sustainable excellence in the healthcare industry.

The question that rings out loud is, "How do we transform our traditional culture to meet the demands of healthcare reform." Clarity and agreement is amiss among healthcare stakeholders on the best steps to take to reach this transformation.

The Culture Cure lays the organizational foundational values to support a culture of excellence. Authentic culture transformation must originate with the people who work within the organization. Culture Transformation begins in an organization when we begin to thoughtfully examine the core organizational values and how colleagues/employees interrelate in the work environment. Do the core values support excellence? Just as individuals have the opportunity to change themselves on the inside, an organization has this privilege. People are where they are, because of the way they think, and if they do not like where they are, then they have the free will to change the way they are thinking.

The healthcare industry will ultimately be healed by the healthcare workers that have dedicated their lives toward the healing of mankind. As innovated and strong healthcare leaders of the 21st century, our job is to reengineer and develop the BEST healthcare delivery system in the world.

Laying fertile foundational ground for cultural transformation takes effort and cannot be taken for granted. There may be an eagerness for transformation steps to be gleamed over, but omission of any of these foundational steps will jeopardize sustainability of culture excellence in an organization. Attempting to pass over the establishment of core values will lead the efforts of cultural transformation process into a "flavor of the month" or "shooting star initiative" within the organization. This taste dissipates quickly and the star will land ultimately on the side of a culture that does not heal, but hurts.

Ignoring environmental culture factors and their importance will continue to propel a poorly functioning healthcare system. A new valued-based healthcare culture of the future will be proactive in preventing the fall of Humpty Dumpty.

The Culture Cure took root within my heart and soul from working in the healthcare industry as a Radiologic Technologist, Educator, Manager, Director, Vice President and CEO over 35 years. I have a deep passion for the people who dedicate their lives to improving the health and well-being of others, and made it my personal mission to create, maintain, and sustain a transcendent culture within healthcare environments. This book represents the core foundational principles that support the infrastructure for my Corporate Transcendence™ Curriculum that is not included in this book. The seed for this culture transformation curriculum took root in my being over 20 years ago.

Over a period of 16 years, I had the opportunity to test portions of my Corporate Transcendence™ curriculum in hospital settings, and then the opportunity came to put the completed curriculum to the test, under the most challenging and devastating organizational circumstances possible over a 6 year period. The outcomes resulted in excellence in organizational culture, patient quality, governance, and financial viability. This self-help book is the open door to required preparation an organization must take in order to prepare the way for transcendence, which means taking an organization continually above and beyond excellence.

The Core Foundational Principles represented by this book along with the Corporate Transcendence™ Transformational Curriculum grew organically from the healthcare industry, but it is also applicable to other industries represented in the following sectors:

* Schools or school systems, community colleges, universities
* Nonprofits and government organizations, local, state, and federal
* Service organizations, including faith-based organizations
* Manufacturing
* Small Business

The foundational principles and curriculum is also scalable and sizable to organizations. This cross over from healthcare to other industry is similar to quality management system in the 1968, known as Total Quality Management (TQM). TQM is the name for a broad and systemic approach to managing organizational quality. Kaoru Ishikawa's synthesis of the philosophy contributed to Japan's ascension as a world quality leader. Corporate Transcendence™ represented a broad integrated systemic tool that supports culture (work environment), quality (patient care), finance (profitability) and governance (regulatory standards) to achieve excellence. Similar to TQM, Corporate Transcendence™ – CT prepares an organization to be the top in its global industry sector. Malcolm Baldrige Excellence Award speaks to many of the principles and processes that comprise CT.

Do No Harm

How we function as healthcare professionals in the patient clinical setting determines whether the patient heals or improves their health outcomes, or experiences health degradation or possible death. In the healthcare industry there has been a desperate need to create a work environment that is conducive to the most immediate results and long term outcomes for the patients. To "do no harm," we must proactively find potential risk within our complex environment of healthcare and be prepared to take appropriate action to reduce them. For those of us that have walked the concrete floors of healthcare for years, this is much easier said than done. An industry that is complex, with a vast number of parts moving at the same time can become dysfunctional quickly. Healthcare professionals speak of the need for standing orders or protocol, that represents an intentional strategic methodology that proactively safeguards against errors and dysfunction.

The Institute of Medicine's landmark report, *To Err is Human: Building a Safer Health System* (1999) revealed that tens of thousands of Americans die every year from medical errors. There is a higher risk for human error to occur when there is an unhealthy work culture.

The healthcare industry and governmental stakeholders desire a better system that fosters the least amount of harm possible. I've written this book that aligns with a Corporate Transcendence™ curriculum for America's healthcare with the ultimate goal of providing a proven model of care, that will provide patients with the best care possible and healthcare workers continued excellence in culture (work environment), quality (patient care), governance (regulatory standards) and finance (profitability). This book is for you if you want the following things:

- You want to know that the healthcare facility you and your loved ones use is a healthy place for people to work, with minimal stress or anxiety.
- You want to use healthcare organizations that foster an environmental culture that values employees.
- You want people who are receiving care to achieve the best possible health results.
- You want patients care to be delivered by happy, committed, accountable caregivers.
- You want patients to have effective management of their disease states, as well as, improved health outcomes and excellent proactive and preventive care.
- You want a culture that heals and not kills in our healthcare systems.

This book will introduce you to these transformative principles as well as many of the effective practices it employs. Follow these principles to create a culture that heals, with engaging and thriving employees, in a profitable organization, that produces best practices in patient care delivery. *The Culture Cure* represents proven and tested leadership and organizational foundational values.

CHANGING TIMES

In 2014, the resignation of the Veterans Administration top health official, Dr. Robert Petzel, followed by the resignation of the Secretary of Veterans Affairs, Eric Shinseki, was a repeat of historical complaints with the government-run Veteran Administration healthcare system. A presidential audit ordered by President Barack Obama concluded that hundreds of thousands of veterans did not receive care in a timely manner or received substandard care. The need for completely new style of innovative leadership to overhaul the government healthcare system was needed, and President Obama final selection of a leader was from outside of the healthcare industry. Robert A. McDonald, previous Chairman, President and CEO of Procter and Gamble took over the largest healthcare system in America to lead this transformation process and became the 8th United States Secretary of Veterans Affairs.

Reviving traditional healthcare to meet the public's approval requires a comprehensive, systemic approach. A complete transfusion for new life is needed. Unfortunately traditional culture remains very entrenched in many cases, and transformation can appear like an insurmountable feat. Leading healthcare organizations that have embraced transformation has shown that it is feasible. The question remains is it sustainable. To achieve sustainability it begins from the ground up to transfuse new blood and life in a new healthcare culture.

Culture eats strategy for breakfast, lunch, and dinner. Because culture can only be expressed through people, culture transformation begins first and foremost with people transformation. For many healthcare entities this means peeling back the existing culture and subcultures in order to rebuild a new culture.

This process reminds me of an interesting story found in Greek history, about the eternal life and majestic transformation of the immortal bird, the Phoenix. The Phoenix, while retiring to its nest at a very old age is literally consumed from the sun's fiery furnace. From ashes, the phoenix undergoes total transformation and is reborn to become once more a magnificent bird with extraordinary beauty, power and strength. The American healthcare industry has the ability to represent excellence, power, and strength again to the world, just like the Phoenix rising from the ashes.

This book is a direct result of many experiences and lessons I have learned while in my healthcare career journey as an educator, middle manager, senior leader, and turnaround CEO. Once heard that an author creates the world in which they desire to live. This statement holds truth for me. Culture is an extremely broad subject. One book could never come close to serving justice to the topic. In this book, I pass along proven truths as a guide to support my colleagues as they work to deliver the best healthcare system possible. It will be through partnering and sharing our best practices with a servant mindset, that American healthcare leaders will successfully lead, and healthcare employees will successfully swim the waters of landmark change back to the best healthcare system in the world.

The Culture Cure provides foundational principles for continuous cultural transformation to excellence and beyond. A Cultural Work Environment assessment is provided in the back of this book and is also provided free at www.CorporateTranscendence.com. This assessment survey tool will assist in determining the true culture of an organization. It was my desire, for this book not to be about the restatement of industry problems, but to share as many possible application opportunities that this reading would allow. Among the chapters you will see many best practices that have been tested and at the end of Chapters 4-12 there are Action Steps dedicated to the Front Line, Management, and Leadership. Also provided are applicable Value Symbols that can be used to recognize and reward colleagues that exhibits the core foundational principles of Vision, Leadership, Ownership, Personal Strengths, Equipping, Empowerment, Momentum, and Success.

Becoming a Transformational Leader

My experience from many years in healthcare left me feeling that as leaders we had been reacting to the demands of payers in our industry to a degree that it dominated our leadership and management behaviors. The payers defined our organizational identities and cultivated in our organizations strong self-limiting beliefs. As healthcare leaders we believed if we could keep the payers happy, we could and would exist indefinitely. That is the typical business world mindset, but based on the fact that healthcare is the only industry that cares for illnesses and trauma to people many times without payment, and the reimbursement system of third party payers is unique as compared to other business. To survive in healthcare it takes more than a retail mentality.

This mindset limited creative and innovative thinking in actual patient care. Status quo appeared fine as long as we were getting paid. New service line business plans had to have strong attachments to the bottom line. In my years as a senior leader in healthcare service line development, I was constantly scanning the horizon for new services and technology opportunities tied to what the commercial, Medicare, and Medicaid payers would allow in payment to enhance our organizations bottom line. A healthy bottom line was the main objective, justified by the fact that this would provide more services locally for our patients. It was definitely a mindset of diagnosing and treating versus prevention. With additional services and equipment procurement, the bottom line gained additional revenue, based on higher-cost to payers and patients.

As a member of the senior leadership, I had to have confidence that the hospital had all the bells and whistles to provide better patient care and receive greater reimbursement. Patient care and access was priority. My struggle however, was with the hospital's financial challenges precipitated by a community that could not afford these services. This is often the thoughts for healthcare leaders across America. Healthcare leaders struggle with the balancing act of offering the best they can in healthcare to all people, and still remain financially sound.

In addition, I repeatedly observed that the healthcare work climate seemed chaotic, drowning in rapid changing expectations and demands. Employees were expected to adjust and acclimate like superheroes. By default, this command control environment seemed justifiable by necessity and time constraints. Numerous time-limited employee meetings to distribute more stacks of new and revised policies for compliance, created an education system that was like drinking from a fire hose. Employees were expected to quickly become both experts and enforcers of policy while continuing to perform their job with compassion and a smile. Among leadership, our mindset assumed that since most healthcare employees earned professional degrees, they should be able to function effectively under continuous, high demands. Should not health professional be willing to accept this environment since they opted to be part of the industry? From this paradox, I witnessed a culture that may have contributed to the death of a young patient, through the inherent complexities of our healthcare environment. That day was a final wake up call, and it became a mental, as well as a soulful crossroad for me. No longer could I sit back to accept the status quo of healthcare.

The accepted commander control, hierarchical leadership and management culture so evident across the healthcare landscape created a lot of internal conflict and pain for me. I developed great empathy for overworked, overburdened healthcare workers that would never intentionally do harm. Their desire to care and serve people encouraged them to pursue a career in healthcare. Unfortunately, like me, they discovered that coping with a complex dysfunctional system required major survival skills and living through episodes of personal burnout.

Through my accumulation of diverse work experiences, I was deeply motivated to begin my personal quest to discover the secret formula to reinvent our healthcare culture. I desired to develop a healthy culture that would exceed our patient's expectations, meet all the regulatory guidelines, have happy and high performing employees, and provide a healthy financial bottom line. After reading every book I could find on healthcare culture, I realized that most discussions focused on what was wrong with the culture; and provided very few insights of knowledge on how to fix it.

A more current process mapping company that at that time, my hospital struggled with patient satisfaction scores as low as single digits. In fact, it took three years for leadership and management to believe that the problem may be the organization and not with the patients that completed the survey. Sound familiar?

While a member of the C-Suite, struggling with this unhealthy culture, I signed on to a three year commitment to help lead and teach an employee customer service program. It took this length of time to ensure each employee attended the education once. The program focused on the frontline employees, because they were the ones who were thought to have the greatest influence on the patient's experience. The program did offer a few components of personal development, again for the employees only. Management and leadership entered the training to do Q &A only. Administration had specific goals around this program: employees would have better attitudes, morale would improve, and patient satisfaction scores would increase. The "we-they" mentality remained entrenched. The majority of employees gave the program high scores, with the exception of one department that administration labeled as "the troublemakers." It seemed the staff only wanted to talk about the things wrong in their department. Although the program was declared successful by leadership and our patient satisfaction showed minimal positive response, this short-lived improvement did not bring consistency or a long-term solution to improve customer service. I decided, instead of ignoring those "troublemakers," I would engage them to better understand the source of their dissatisfaction. I learned firsthand that we needed to develop a comprehensive systemic plan instead of rehashing a two day customer service "feel good" program.

The next approach was to create an organic, in-house customer service program. We created a cross-sectional team of leaders to focus on this goal. This approach brought about some success; however these wins did not result in a significant increase in patient satisfaction scores and consistent improvement in patient quality outcomes.

In searching for answers we engaged a customer service company that specialized in improving patient satisfaction scores by focusing on frontline engagement and empowerment. In a few months we saw noticeable changes and patient satisfaction began to improve. However, sustainability faltered due to lack of consistent engagement of leadership in the program. As support from the C-Suite evaporated, the initiative died shortly thereafter. Over the following years I continued to organically experiment with cultures and subcultures with a goal of creating the initiative that has eventually become a successful comprehensive curriculum of excellence.

In 2009, I found myself with the opportunity to become the Chief Executive Officer of a large community healthcare system that was literally on the brink of bankruptcy. Cash flow was in deficient with payroll not being met.

As the new CEO, I took the reins of a community healthcare system that served five counties and offered medical, dental, behavioral health and specialty services. The organization serviced a large uninsured population and individuals who had very limited primary care options. The organization was over $8 million in debt, with a budget of approximately $15 million. The future looked bleak. A visiting Joint Commission surveyor remarked that the organization was essentially "burnt to the ground." Rapid growth and difficulty in reimbursement had played a major role in the organization's financial decline.

Based on my success and failures through the years in development of a culture of excellence in a hospital setting, I knew this organization would serve as the perfect research environment to test my Corporate Transcendence™ curriculum for healthcare excellence. This environment would serve as the testing ground for the culmination of my past experiences. I realized there was a great need to refocus employee attention on what they could be empowered to do, instead of being consumed with the daily experience of working in a financially devastated organization. The organization's rallying cry became "We will not fail."

At the same time I was bailing water in financial distress, I immediately brought in Custom Learning Healthcare from Calgary, Canada to help begin the process improving customer service in a depressed environment. They refocused staff onto aspects of the organization they could change and as the CEO; I focused on restructuring and rebuilding the culture, quality, finance, and governance of the organization. My colleagues, the Board of Directors and I along with external cultural and financial support slowly repaired and began to rebuild the organization.

Good news! After approximately three years, the organization financially stabilized and I knew it was time to take over complete ownership of our workplace culture, and develop a core that would continue to grow, innovate, and propel the organization forward. We were able to engage our incredible colleagues using nine foundational principles to excel in all areas of operations. Through the implementation of the Corporate Transcendence™ curriculum that affected every area of the organization (culture, quality, finance, and governance) and investments into personal and professional growth for all staff; the employees became positively motivated, more engaged and empowered. The foundation for a highly reliable healthcare organization emerged.

Over the next 2 years, the organization was functioning with a solid Corporate Transcendence™ curriculum that engaged and empowered frontline colleagues, healthcare providers, middle management, and senior leadership. Team and collaborative leadership were practiced at all levels. The curriculum created a transparency, along with a learning questioning knowledge based environment that was not satisfied with stagnant operations, but intentionally sought constant improvement in all services.

The culture had made the transformation to a culture proactively searching for improvements, enjoying success, and expecting excellence in all work. Employees became colleagues. Valuing each colleague, identifying and utilizing their strengths increased the value of the organization. Internal promotions and succession planning for positions progressed naturally.

We intentionally referred to each other as colleagues instead of employees to further model our team leadership model at all levels of the organization. Employee is defined as a person who works for another person or a business for pay. Colleague is someone that you work with or alongside. Using "colleague" when referring to a co-worker was decided for all employees regardless of title or position to show sensitivity in valuing each person and their strengths in the organization. I suggest this best practice as a consideration in your organization.

Patient, employee and provider satisfaction improved drastically. Financial revenue enhancement was significant. In just five years the organization showed no resemblance to its previous toxic, dying culture. It was thriving, financially sound, and continuously moving to significant improvements in quality, culture, finance, and governance. The expectation of excellence in all areas became the guiding principle of daily work. The empowering movement of a positive culture became familiar, expected and enjoyed! Accolades of winning annual national service excellence awards became the norm and quality outcomes for patient care received national recognition.

The Corporate Transcendence™ curriculum provided the infrastructure for continued excellence to grow across the organization in the medical, dental, behavioral health and specialty departments. The organization adopted the mantra that our excellence tomorrow was better than our excellence today. Progressive annual improvements were demonstrated in the employee and provider satisfaction survey, patient satisfaction survey, patient quality measures, national awards and recognitions for best practices were received, clean financial audits, accreditations through The Joint Commission for Ambulatory and Behavioral Healthcare and Patient Centered Medical Home, and successful Health Resources and Service Administration surveys. The evidence-based documentation of Corporate Transcendence™ success throughout the organization in culture, finance, quality, and governance was further evident in the receiving of the North Carolina Governor's First Milestone Malcolm Baldrige Quest for Excellence award. Our organization achieved this prestigious award during six short years of transformation, progressing the organization from edge of bankruptcy to excellence.

Everything discussed in this book leads back to the first priority of organizational culture development. In my many years working in thriving and failing healthcare organizations, I have realized that culture is the heart of the health of our healthcare industry. This book is my way of valuing America's healthcare system and my healthcare colleagues. My hope is together we can embrace a culture transformation on to excellence and transcendence I commemorate the current and future accomplishments of my colleagues to making the American healthcare model the best in the world. I look forward to partnering with you.

CHAPTER 1

Let the Journey Begin: Diagnosing Healthcare

• • •

"A journey of a thousand miles begins with a single step."

LAO TZU

Diagnosing the root cause of the many issues surrounding healthcare in America has proven to be a major challenge. There is a monumental struggle with diagnosing the underlying sickness and finding a treatment plan that will be comprehensive enough to eradicate all its ailments. The symptoms of overpriced care, financially stretched organizations, stressed and disillusioned providers and healthcare workers, unhealthy patient outcomes, and in many cases minimal standards of care create a complex, dysfunctional condition. There is yet to be a maximum strength medication manufactured to cure the symptoms for the over challenged state of healthcare in America. Because healthcare is the lifeline to the quality of life and longevity of all Americans, everyone seems to have an opinion. Politicians and the media have a lot to say about the state of healthcare in America, but the solutions seem to be scarce.

Why is determining a diagnosis and finding a cure for healthcare so challenging? When healthcare providers diagnose a sickness, we assess the symptoms and obtain a personal history to see if there is a link to the sickness. The symptoms reveal that healthcare in America is weakened, not life-saving, but in some cases life-threatening. Among 11 western countries, the United States healthcare system is one of the most expensive in the world and ranks last for efficiency, equity and outcomes according to the Commonwealth Fund.[i]

How can this happen? The United States is often perceived as "the land of plenty" for nourishment and a quality lifestyle. Healthcare is a significant part of the social infrastructure and cannot be ignored by any country that desires to be viable and strong socially and economically. In the United States, great emphasis has been placed on healthcare as it represent a country that values human life in many ways. Many aspects of life of an individual or a country depend on a people being healthy and free of disease. In the very essence of our society, healthcare is a central core component of America's landscape.

A Sick Heart

When there are abnormal symptoms of a vital organ such as the heart, there is grave concern. The heart is a life-sustaining organ. A poorly functioning heart can quickly become life-threatening and requires immediate attention, often drastic measures. Healthcare is a vital component, arguably the heart, of any country. Without a properly functioning healthcare system, there will be major sickness and disease, epidemics, and preventable deaths.

Addressing problems found in healthcare will require stakeholders to understand the strategic departure and arrival points, and identify what components will provide the greatest influence for success. What is clear today is if we continue to follow past thinking, we cannot expect things to change.

Our Reality Check

As healthcare leaders and stakeholders, we need to come into agreement that there are many opportunities for improvement. Even more importantly, we must hold ourselves accountable. We cannot become aware of the solutions we need, if we ignore truths. Blaming and pointing fingers for the state of America's healthcare is no better than burying our heads in the sand hoping all our problems will go away. Unfortunately there is no single silver bullet to fix healthcare. But that does not mean it cannot be transformed and become the model of choice in the world again. The problems of healthcare are ours to solve, and the best solutions will come from our own pool of healthcare professionals.

CURE NEEDED

To cure the American healthcare system, we need continuous innovation and enlightenment coming from our colleagues and leadership. We must find new ways to bring continuous excellence to our system. This task calls for visionaries, risk takers, and critical thinkers. It will require compassion, values-based leadership, empathy, personal and professional development, accountability, empowerment, engagement, and teamwork. With the information contained in this book, you can join the evidence-based courageous pioneers who are willing to reject status quo healthcare and create a culture that continuously delivers excellence in every way.

PARTNERING FOR SUCCESS

Effective collaboration is an indispensable part of the healthcare cure. It necessitates creating open communication, and collaboration, utilizing innovative practices like roundtables for all stakeholders to guide the process. Crippling gaps have to be closed. For example, gaps in the mission alignment of healthcare organizations and the academia teachings of healthcare students, gaps between employees, providers and leadership and governance. Every stakeholder needs to be at the table to own and be accountable to the future of healthcare in America.

21ST CENTURY HEALTHCARE

The traditional world of healthcare is quickly becoming irrelevant. Now is the time to heal healthcare through culture transformation. Many factors in the healthcare industry are forcing healthcare organizations to engage the patient in a holistic way – physically, emotionally, behaviorally, and through social determinants. The same holistic approach delivers powerful results when used with the healthcare colleague – from frontline staff to leadership. When patients are engaged in healthcare, they become more accountable and responsible to meet their personal healthcare needs, and are on their way to improved health. The same holds true of a healthcare colleague. When colleagues are engaged and empowered, they become more accountable and responsible for their actions. Colleagues become engaged when they know they are valued and their opinions are respected. This cultivates innovative thinking and supports personal ownership of the organization's future.

INTERDEPENDENCE

The future or sustainable healthcare organizations must be free of silos or islands. All stakeholders are interdependent on each other for success. The functional missions of all major stakeholders are unique to some degree, but the culture of one environment cannot conflict with the other. Unifying signals and messages that are consciously and unconsciously communicated to our healthcare student, providers, colleagues, and patients must be in alignment for a harmonious work environment and best outcome for the patient. All stakeholders must agree and be willing to make any and all adjustments in academia, cultures, thoughts, and behavior to obtain this.

NEW AGE

In the new age of healthcare, our goal of improving population health is best supported by meeting people where they are. This means taking a holistic view of the person, taking in consideration the social determinants of the patient's health. It requires helping people through education, and providing the appropriate resources to put the patient in the driver's seat, to help them arrive at a place of improved health. By doing this, we empower the whole person and help them to not only treat the disease, but to build health and wellness. The same applies to developing a culture that heals versus a culture that kills. We need to have a cultural determinant for cultural health in organizations. Transforming your culture into one which fosters healthy outcomes for the organization is vital. Engaging and empowering healthcare colleagues is the essential link to developing a culture that will sustain public scrutiny in healthcare today, and meet the needs that traditional healthcare could not.

ECHOING CRY

Across the country, Americans are speaking out for change, seeking a healthcare system that can meet their needs. How will healthcare leaders make the large scale changes to thrive in an environment marked by landmark legislation like the arrival of the Patient Protection and Affordable Care Act? Facing a population that has an escalating need for care, how can the 12 million men and women who currently work in the healthcare industry in the United States remain committed to what they do and flourish in the new age of healthcare? *The Culture Cure* provides the solid foundation to support leaders in meeting the challenges of an innovative and transformed healthcare system. If you do not have an innovative, transformed healthcare organization, this book will provide the guidance needed to begin organizational transcendence.

A BLUEPRINT

My experience has shown that organizations need to have an internal development curriculum blueprint, but many organizations fail to seek this or adopt one. Corporate Transcendence™ curriculum creates a platform which allows employees to continue to expand and develop their abilities, and stretch themselves for personal growth. An organization which does this will support organic employee retention and succession. It should be a budgeted priority for the organization, due to its tremendous financial return on investment and pay off for the organization in culture, quality, and governance. A transcendent organization is grown within colleagues by building their personal competence, character, and relationships and influence with others. It is a smoother succession for the organization to promote colleagues from within who know the values and culture of the organization. Growing expertise within keeps a culture in more optimal health helps the bottom line, provides more consistent quality of care, and provides a less risk for governance by affecting internal regulatory hardwiring.

UNLEASHING EXCELLENCE

When you have connected to your truths and values – and have built influence-based leadership – it is time to unleash excellence within your organization. To do this you have to release people at every level of the organization, and allow them to grow. Unleashing excellence is achieved by establishing a strong foundation of culture, quality, finance, and governance that I will refer to often in this book as the Four Cornerstones of Healthcare which we will discuss further in subsequent chapters. (I also refer to these as the Four Trees of Transcendence in my Corporate Transcendence™ curriculum, but for simplicity and understanding, I chose to use terms more commonly heard.)

Natural unleashing of colleague's positive characteristics and behaviors can abound, and open transparency and accountability can become the conscious and subconscious of the organization. People are challenged, engaged, empowered, confident, and competent to continuously improve the organization.

When true excellence germinates, it flows from ALL people within the organization. Everyone is a stakeholder and everyone has a role in creating and living in the excellence zone each and every day. One team's success becomes a win for the entire organization. Teaching colleagues to praise jobs well done and to eagerly value the team's efforts fosters trust and creates a supportive culture. It is only in this kind of culture that each individual can own their place in the organization, and actively participate in creating sustainable excellence. The level of engagement creates a stakeholders mindset. True stakeholders have a voice; we must give all colleagues a voice if we want engagement from them. Giving a voice to colleagues empowers them as owners of the organization. Colleagues influence in creating innovation and fresh thinking strengthens the organization in every way.

A remarkable transformation occurs when the colleague stakeholder's creative mindset permeates the organization. Leaders empower colleagues to contribute to innovation, and excellence follows. This happens when transformational thinking becomes automatic and a habit in the subconscious. An organization that achieves this level of transformational thinking transcends the traditional healthcare mindset and has the power to overcome the enormous challenges in healthcare today. Healthcare colleagues thrive. Transformation can heal healthcare in America. Let's do it together.

ACTION STEPS

At the end of nine of the chapters, you will find recommendations for actions. The "Frontline Culture Transformation Steps" can be taken by colleagues with non-management roles in an organization. "Management Culture Transformation Steps" are designed for any colleague in a managerial or team leadership role. "Executive Culture Transformation Steps" are those that require the highest level of responsibility and decision-making influence.

VALUES SYMBOLS OF EXCELLENCE

There are nine value symbols taught within this book. They represent core foundational values that support organizational excellence that are needed to build a culture of transcendence. These symbols are designed to communicate excellence and encourage and recognize colleagues that embrace their meaning through their behavior. Using this recognition in your organization will contribute to a culture that fosters vision, leadership, empathy, ownership, personal strengths, momentum, equipping, empowerment, and success.

CHAPTER 2

Value of Valuing:
The Nonnegotiable Step

• • •

*"The act of valuing others is the greatest
gift you can give yourself."*

MORGAN HENDRIX

Connecting and having a positive relationship with colleagues should be the golden thread that runs through an organization. Trust, integrity, service, compassion, respect, and excellence are powerful values that are at the center of vibrant healthcare organizations. But there is a single core value that is the bedrock for all of the others. We will label this *core value* as "valuing others." This value is about intentionally opening our minds and hearts to appreciate our colleagues and the patients we serve. The essence of connecting through valuing requires a level of sensitivity to human existence and the emotional signals that people vibrate. Regardless of the core values adopted in a healthcare organization, valuing others is vital as we represent an industry of healing arts, caring, and service to human beings. Valuing is the bedrock for core organizational values, just like trust is to integrity.

The valuing core competency must be grounded in order to build a solid foundation for cultural excellence. Valuing must be established to leverage the ability to connect with others. Valuing should be expected and easily identified by others. If you do not have positive valuing and live accordingly every day, the organization's mission and vision reality will be at risk. This makes valuing a crucial priority for all leadership positions. Never underestimate the value of valuing people.

Aligning Personal and Corporate Values

The behavior of your colleagues – from the top executive to the front-line employee – reveals what values are being lived. This means leadership and governing boards have the responsibility of establishing and embracing values and expectations, and must lead and mirror the values being lived within the organization. Values should intentionally be set by leadership and not taken for granted as a paper exercise. Values are vetted daily in organizations by people's behavior. For example, people have to know the organization fosters and exhibits the core value of valuing in order to have effective communication and efficient day-to-day interactions.

Remember the impact of personal values on your organization. We cannot assume that honesty and integrity are part of a candidate's personal values when recruiting top leadership and board members for organizations. A values assessment can be vital to the interview process for executive leadership, board members and for all employees to ensure personal values and the organizational values align. People can profess convincingly in interviewing opportunities that they have integrity, but their past and future actions and attitude may tell a more reliable story. As in everything, "Your walk talks louder that your talk talks."

A strategy for assessing a candidate's "walk" for values alignment should be developed and applied before bringing new employees and soon to be colleagues into your organization. Consider ongoing review of these values with colleagues to ensure everyone remains on the same page. Core organizational values will frame the operations and daily functions and an annual evaluation of these values with colleagues is suggested to ensure everyone is living the values. Over time, values will rest in the subconscious state of the organization. Just like a human has subconscious values established by experience conditioning in their life, so too will a well-led organization.

VALUES AND WORK ENVIRONMENT

The personal values – good or bad – are embedded in every person that becomes employed by the organization. These values contribute to having a healing environment, or a toxic one. It requires intentional leadership to create an environment that has positive values. Healthy organizational values equate with healthy personal values. Positive values create a positive personal energy that brings vibrancy to an organization. It is important to recognize that if the values we want in our organization are not being modeled on a personal level, then the organizational values will slip and undesired values will begin to surface.

Values can create an environment of function or dysfunction in an organization. What values do you see on display among our healthcare environment? Traditional healthcare has fostered silos in departments and information. This often manifests such values as separateness, independence, entitlement, and distrust. Highly dysfunctional environments spring from toxic values like dishonesty, self-preservation, and apathy. Vibrant environments grow from healthy values such as teamwork, trust, empathy, ownership, empowerment, and authenticity.

One huge factor in fostering healthy values into the work environment is recognizing that values are just as important in the relationship and behaviors of colleagues to one another, as they are between colleagues and patients. Staff members need to feel caring, respect, and a sense of worth as much as patients do. Organizational values do not discriminate; they cannot apply to one group and not to the entire work population. Because of their impact, we hold values sacred to the culture. We live and guard them as the powerful, success-defining truths that they are. Values are housed in colleagues and contribute greatly to success. They should be factored into our recruitment efforts, patient care and the day-to-day interactions between healthcare colleagues.

CONNECTING PIECES FOR CULTURE CHANGE

Positive values connect people. In healthcare we see this work among colleagues and in the patient-caregiver relationship. For example, empathy is a great value that helps people to be more sensitive to each other. A caregiver becomes more sensitive to a patient by seeking to understand the patient's world perspective. This requires cultural competency and developing an awareness and appreciation of the patient's emotions.

The same is true for showing empathy for a colleague diagnosed with breast cancer, or who faces multiple personal challenges at home. Embracing the value of empathy makes us strive to understand the individual circumstances and challenges, and enables us to treat them with more care and compassion. Empathy as a value demonstrates an emotional bond which creates a connection with another person. Every other positive value also creates moments of connectedness between people within the culture – trust, accountability, excellence, leadership, teamwork. Every value builds a type of connectivity when we put them into action. Connection created through positive values grows deeper personal connections. They make an organization more successful by having happier employees who feel appreciated, valued, and understood.

Connecting allows for opening up and greater transparency to others. Genuine connecting happens when real or perceived barriers come down and there is a safe environment with flowing dialogue. Connecting is fundamental to trust. Trust is a result of a human connection or exchange that has gone well. Connection is impossible without trust. When trust is lost, the communication and relationship deteriorates.

CHAPTER 3

Leadership and Values: Alignment Matters

• • •

"Example is not the main thing in influencing others. It is the only thing."

ALBERT SCHWEITZER

LEADING WITH INFLUENCE

Many times there is a perception or belief that if a person can obtain a leadership title that they will instantly become a successful person of influence. Leadership titles do not improve a person's ability to lead. The leaders then define for themselves if they are a great leaders or the type of leader they are or will become. History has proven that many people have been promoted or given a title, but proved to be very poor or weak leaders. A title is positioning – nothing more, nothing less. Being a great leader requires competence, character, and the ability to connect with and influence others.

LEADING WITH COMPETENCE

Leadership is providing the vision, clarity, and influence to move people forward. Competence is needed in order for others to listen to and or engage with leaders. That is why preparation for leadership roles is necessary and important. No one can just open a great leader's head and drop in the competence, character, interpersonal skills, and influence needed to be a great leader. It takes considerable time, years of practice, energy, sacrifice, focus, commitment and numerous other characteristics to become a great leader. Appropriate education and continuous learning, mingled with life and leadership experiences, are key to being a great leader who effectively influences others.

Competence reveals itself in everything the leader does, including the way they handle mistakes. Admitting and reflecting on wrong decisions in order to learn and grow is part of being a competent leader. A leader who demonstrates the value of "failing forward" increases their influence. Great leaders live out their positive character attributes, rather than just talking about them. With or without a title, if you have influence, you are a leader. Be conscious of your attitudes and behaviors, and develop your leadership skills. Build your influence through demonstrating competence and character. This builds respect for your opinions, and strengthens your voice, and supports the organization and administration in many positive ways during organizational changes including culture transformation.

When I say that any healthcare colleague can have great influence, it is because it is true for every person. Think of Mother Teresa. Her massively influential life began working as a nun without a special title or position of authority. Over time she gained the respect of the world and connected with millions of people, and was able to influence some of the most distinguished and powerful people in the world. Every person should think of themselves as a leader, even if the only person they are influencing is them self. People who desire to be a leader should have an understanding that first they must exercise self-leadership before leading others effectively can ever be possible.

ENLARGING YOUR CIRCLE OF INFLUENCE

The circle of influence analogy is great to illustrate that if a person works effectively within their own job responsibilities or circle, it is normally noticed by others. The more effectively they carry out their job, the more they are recognized by leaders and the greater their circle of influence will become. This can often lead to promotions, increased compensation, and new job opportunities. The key here is to concentrate on what you can control and the job responsibilities that you are supposed to do. Do not fall into the habit of worrying about other people and their jobs. Focus on your role and your responsibilities and the performance of your job will be noticed. People are given jobs for a reason and if the job was not needed they would not be there. Focus on your job, as it affects the entire company, and perform the very best you can. You will then earn your paycheck for a job well done. Your colleagues and associates will notice your efforts.

I encourage you to perform with excellence in your personal circle of influence and continue to learn and grow yourself professionally. Adapt and maintain positive leadership values and people skills along the way. These actions place you on the track to become an influential person and a great leader.

Great leaders must possess and continually develop their people skills. Intentionally staying in touch with the needs and work being performed by colleagues within the organization is as important as attending a board meeting. Great leaders seek to keep the pulse of the organization near them, in order to aid them in the navigation of the vision of the organization.

Many people have been promoted to leadership positions based on their competence, but did not possess good people skills. Without relationship skills they will continue to lose influence among all stakeholders. A promotion based solely on a colleague's popularity is as dangerous as promoting a colleague beyond their competencies or abilities.

A leader has to possess people skills to be able to influence others. Influence will not prevail if there is tension and conflict. Developing future healthcare leaders is an important responsibility of organizational leadership, just as much as the educational institutions. Some healthcare organizations have supported college tuition in targeted healthcare fields due to shortages, or as part of an employee benefit package. This is great to some degree, if the budget permits; but there are other options to promote employees to enhance their skills, talents, and education which have a much greater payoff for organizational excellence and success. A colleague personal and professional internal growth curriculum is a great place to begin.

CHAPTER 4

Directive Vision:
Destination of Excellence

• • •

*"A vision is not just a picture of what could be; it is an appeal
to our better selves, a call to become something more."*

ROSABETH MOSS KANTER

DEFINING VISION

Vision is the overarching goals and aerial view of the future. It is not
only who we are, but also who we are trying to become. Vision brings
hope for a better way, a greater day, and a hope for good things. People
get inspired by vision. When we cast a positive vision and then keep
it constantly in front of us, it will inspire us to keep moving on the
path and to make a difference. If we lose our vision we lose our hope.
When we lose hope we lose our reason to be. Mission is what you DO.
Vision is what you aspire to Become. We have to remember that vision
is meaningless unless people can comprehend and see it. Every leader
must continually cast and bring the vision into daily operational reality.
A clear vision has power. It should become your organizations mantra.

The following is an analogy to the importance of having vision.

THE STORY OF THE WOOD SCULPTOR

There was an accomplished wood sculptor who saw a large tree trunk lying on the farm of a large plantation property owner. He inquired of the owner what his intention was for the cut trees. The plantation owner told him that he had no use for the huge logs, and would probably burn or destroy them. The sculptor asked the owner if he could have the discarded wood and the owner agreed.

The sculptor hauled large pieces of wood home. The next day he cut a large piece of wood and stood the tall piece of wood up on its trunk end. He began to walk slow circles around and around the wood, pausing at times as he continued to scan the tree trunk from top to bottom. After some time had passed, the sculptor took his axe and began to chop at the piece of wood. He chopped repeatedly and made significant cuts into the wood that seem to make no sense or reason. Hours passed and the work continued for several more days.

In the weeks ahead, the plantation owner was passing the wood sculptor's home and saw a magnificent sculpted eagle with its wings spread wide in his yard. It was one of the most beautiful sculptures he had ever seen. He pulled over and eagerly asked his neighbor if he would consider selling the beautiful wooden eagle statue. The sculptor agreed to sell it for five hundred dollars. The plantation owner was delighted and agreed, and they began to load the beautiful eagle onto his truck. The new owner asked his friend how he created the beautiful sculpture. The wood sculptor explained that he never saw dead wood when he asked to have the trees from the plantation owner's house. He said that he immediately saw the vision of something beautiful in the wood. The plantation owner was shocked to hear that the beautiful eagle statue actually came from his cut trees, the wood he had planned to destroy.

Vision begins in the soul's eye. Vision, like most things in life, can be created to be a positive or negative future reality.

VISION MATTERS

Visionaries see something where others see nothing. They can envision the journey and the end in the mind's eye before the vision is cast or the journey begins. Potential victories on the journey and potential barriers are usually already weighed out and addressed. Thomas Edison's discovery of light is a great example of visionary thinking. He saw the outcome no one else saw, as well as the potential path to get there.

Where would people be in this world without vision? So much of our existence and identity as people depend on our visionaries. Freedom, clean water, health cures, equality, healthcare for people, information technology, entrepreneurship, and an endless list of positive realities represent the fruits of vision.

You may recall a time when you were in a meeting and it seemed to be going nowhere and little was accomplished. You may have been in an organization where you did not have a clue about its strategic vision. Much like a flounder out of water, the meeting and the organization flap and move around without direction, unsure of how to get back into the water to remain vibrant in its life. Hopefully, you have also experienced meetings that had clear agendas and purpose, moving participants forward in a directive way. Just like a productive meeting with a purposeful agenda, there needs to be a clear, directive vision for an organization. The daily mission of the organization provides purpose, but without an aerial view of its future, the organization will have no direction to propel itself and prosper. Vision planning and strategic planning go hand in hand. Organizations that do not have a clear, directive vision are much like nomads moving from place to place without a goal for the future. They may be living out their daily mission statement, but there is a stagnant culture where colleagues merely exist in the present moment. This dangerous mindset will not create a healthy environment or culture for the organization. Organizations in today's world cannot stay unchanged with the many external influences in society, businesses, government and the world.

Good leaders realize that vision has to continue to change over time and be continually developed among colleagues in order for the organization to remain successful in the future. Without a vision the people perish. No vision leads to disappointment. Stagnant organizations will stall, driving the organization into a downward spiral instead of a positive upward thrust.

Vision Development

Traditionally, vision statements are designed by senior leaders in partnership with the governing board and a few select staff. Healthcare leaders are expected by community stakeholders and employees to set vision and lead their organization into the future. Today there is an opportunity for a new form of vision planning in healthcare, as healthcare moves toward a team-based leadership model that supports the patient-centric care. Vision is a powerful attribute to have, but does not have to be limited to the traditional handful of leaders. Healing healthcare will require bringing the vision planning to involve individuals at all levels of the organization.

Expanding the opportunity for input from others for vision, or gleaming organizational vision from all healthcare stakeholders in an organization certainly has its appeal. The individuals who do the daily work are the largest vested group of people in the healthcare system. Giving colleagues a chance to weigh in and have a voice provides many different perspectives, insights, and ownership to creating a new vision model. Involvement of colleagues as stakeholders also increases the likelihood of success in vision implementation. It provides greater engagement, ownership, and empowerment for future success of strategic initiatives based on the stated vision for the organization.

If our goal is transformation to reach greater excellence in our healthcare organizations, we need to engage colleagues from all areas of the organization in vision projecting, as well as strategic planning.

The vision for healthcare quality within and among the many healthcare organizations in America will need to be driven from within the industry. The people who do the work every day should be first place in creating best practices in quality of care, finance sustainability, work culture, and regulatory governance compliance. The people performing healthcare duties are the ones who are the most passionate, dedicated and have the greatest knowledge and influence in the ultimate outcomes of healthcare. Healthcare stakeholders that make up the industry have much to give and can play a major role in innovation and creation of vision for America's healthcare industry. Many healthcare organizations have recognized this and are involving more of their colleagues in vision setting, strategic planning, and leading the industry in many innovative best practices.

Solo leadership is dying fast. Traditional views of financial success found in continual growth in number of buildings or acquiring more real-estate will not be the main factor in determining success for future organizations. The new thought age of medicine is being built upon the value of the healthcare service that is represented by the improvements and maintenance of patient health outcomes. This is still a bitter pill for many healthcare colleagues to swallow. As healthcare leaders, we can embrace the current pivotal changes in healthcare delivery and choose to lead, or we can remain stuck in tradition and die a slow death. To achieve best clinical patient outcomes, healthcare leaders will need to lead colleagues into collaborative team leadership culture and share the reins of leadership to make healthcare in America the best.

New Healthcare Vision

Our new vision of success rests on achieving significance. Organizations today need to make a difference, not simply seek to amass large bank balances. Significance will mean casting the vision of healthy community for present and future generations to come. Significance will be recognized by healthier people lives and improved patient outcomes, and the reputation of excellence earned by the healthcare industry.

One of the most famous speeches ever written began with the heart and soul of a person who had a vision or dream for a new reality in America. His vision inspired people of all walks of life, regardless of color, ethnicity, or socioeconomic standing. Martin Luther King Jr's "I Have a Dream" was a vision that encouraged many Americans to make the country a better place for all people to live. It is my hope that the hearts and souls of the readers of this book will be stirred and inspired to help create a greater vision for healthcare in America. This vision will be as impactful as Dr. King's vision in improving the quality of people's live and making this world a better place to live.

COLLABORATIVE VISION DEVELOPMENT

Participating collaboratively in the development of the overarching vision of the organization will take investment of time and energy on behalf of leaders and further investment to engage colleagues. To determine the future vision of the organization, leaders and colleagues must be consciously aware of the organization's strength.

A meaningful way to involve employees in helping to cast vision for the organization is to involve them in strategic planning initiatives. The perspectives and opinions of frontline staff, as well as those from all levels of management, create a work environment where all participants have ownership and are engaged to carry the corporate vision forward. It is ideal to also take a step further and get stakeholders from the community to help define the strategic vision of the organization. The public perspective and what is important to the consumer may vary from the internal stakeholders. Gaining this additional layer of input can only strengthen the vision.

CREATING VISION IN YOUR ORGANIZATION

Any vision requires a number of actions to take place in order to come to life. Tactical strategic goals provide the necessary support for the directive vision to be realized. The ownership and accountability of the overarching vision has to be universally shared amongst all employees regardless of title or role.

For clarity and commitment of the directive vision to occur, there must be continuous nurturing of the vision by leadership. The vision must be made applicable to colleagues and their roles. Employees need to understand the impact they make each day in achieving the directive vision for the organization. It takes the entire work community to reach the vision successfully.

Directive vision is like a huge net that is cast over the organization. When cast correctly, the vision will be realized on a daily basis to take the organization to a better place or greater level of success. The vision statement needs to be seen, felt, and referenced to often as part of the culture. The vision becomes ingrained into the fabric of the organization and worn like a badge. Vision may at times seem to get out of focus for colleagues, due to the high level of functionality of their work and healthcare environment. It is leadership's responsibility to be intuitive and develop their "sixth sense" and to lean in closer to their colleagues to open intentional, clear paths to the directive vision of the organization. This is what is referred to as recalibration of the organization to its vision. Remember that recalibration of the arrival point desired and its benefits will again set the navigational compass back on track to success and excellence.

Looking ahead is critical to making progress. Organizations that do not plan for the future usually end up unable to reach their ultimate goals. Lack of vision in today's global market can be a death trap. Vision provides a sense of direction, purpose and hope for betterment for all stakeholders in the organization.

Strategic Planning Potential Pitfalls

Healthcare organizations as well as many other industries, traditionally use the SWOT (Strengths, Weaknesses, Opportunity, Threats) methodology for strategic planning. This planning is often conducted by board members and leadership at a strategic planning retreat. An external facilitator may be employed to help keep the planning on track for completing a three year set of strategic goals. SWOT has been taught in the best universities for many decades and has served organizations well. A fresh look at mission and vision statements and stepping through the strategic process allows leadership an opportunity to brainstorm, discuss, debate, and focus on what they desire the present and future to look like. This process creates a strategic vision for the future that everyone agrees upon. Unfortunately, after a lengthy and costly process, this vision often does not effectively lead the organization. In some cases, the strategic planning becomes an expensive exercise that has no impact on daily activities or long term outcomes.

SHELF LIFE

Certifying and accrediting organizations that survey healthcare organizations will assess the organization on their strategic plan development and will ask to examine the strategic plan the healthcare organization has created and is living. Unfortunately many times after a robust strategic plan is developed, it may become relegated to the bookshelf, rarely revisited by leaders and out of the reach of colleagues. If this is the case, when employees are asked about the vision or what the strategic plan states in regard to the organization, often they are unaware. They consider it something administration manages, and if there is something employees need to know, they will be told.

Many times due to changing and competing priorities, leadership forgets goals and need to refer back to the strategic plan. The leadership and governing board may feel they succeeded in their strategic planning by reviewing and developing a new strategic plan every three to five years, but unless the strategic plan is a living breathing document that aligns with the daily walk and talk of everyone, it becomes another fairly expensive and time consuming paper exercise.

THE WEAKNESS OF SWOT ANALYSIS

Traditional SWOT Analysis looks at Strengths, Weakness, Opportunity, and Threats. But there are some strong drawbacks to using the SWOT technique. The negative elements of SWOT (Weaknesses and Threats) can drain vital organizational energy. We often describe the process of focusing on weaknesses as drowning or like inviting an energy vampire into the planning process. The net effect of focusing on the negative aspects of SWOT representing 50% of the planning methodology (Weaknesses and Threats), essentially negates the other 50% positive aspects (Strengths and Opportunity). This can be illustrated by the equation of (-5) plus 5 = 0. SWOT strategic planning takes away from the positive strengths and opportunities, wasting and draining energy that could be harnessed for positive thoughts and used to focus more on important strategies that will propel the organization in a more sustainable and significant future.

Focusing on strengths and opportunities has a major impact on building the employee morale and self-esteem as well as organizational esteem. Focusing on weaknesses has the opposite effect in most cases. Spending about 5% of an organization's time on weaknesses should suffice. Spending 95% of time on organizational strengths or how to improve upon strengths generates a much greater return in all areas.

APPRECIATIVE INQUIRY AND STRATEGIC PLANNING

One contemporary method that deserves study and attention in the healthcare industry is using Appreciative Inquiry for strategic planning. This method was developed at Case Western Reserve Universities of Cleveland, Ohio Department for Organizational Behavior. The early architects of the Appreciative Inquiry School of thought recognized the inherent flaws in the "problem solving" process; starting with the problem and working toward a solution, bypassing ideas that can innovate, rather than simply repair.

Appreciative Inquiry is gaining more traction among the business and educational industries, framing an organization in a more positive manner for success. Businesses want to focus on what they can be, rather than framing every strategy and decision in light of immediate challenges and deficiencies.

A strategic planning model from the Appreciative Inquiry school of thought is SOAR. This is an alternative to SWOT. SOAR evaluates Strengths, Opportunities, Aspirations, and Results. This method focuses on positive elements in the organization. In theory, focusing on the positive elements and strengths of the organization will diminish the impact of weaknesses over time. In my experience, I have witnessed this theory's success through utilizing the SOAR strategic planning method in healthcare. In my experience, all colleagues participate through department and leadership meetings, along with the community members and the governing board. The process actually built optimism, comradery and enthusiasm among and between all participants. Success seems inevitable, when these collective stakeholder energies focus on strengths, opportunities, aspirations, and results.[ii]

COLLABORATIVE STRATEGIC VISION PLANNING

Collaborative vision planning will demonstrate how insightful employees can be in understanding the organizational needs to succeed in excellence. This reasoning makes sense since colleagues are highly vested, many times spending more than 40 hours per week in the healthcare work environment.

A patient's perspective and voice is invaluable; the patient is invested as the user of the services. It is vital to know if the healthcare organization is meeting the patients' needs or not. Community assessments are valuable factual tools to understand as well. But the advantage in planning for the future comes from the actual boots on the ground, the colleagues. They will give the organization the edge in having the soundest insight for planning for the future of the organization.

Focusing on strengths is a positive initiative for organizations, and it is also valuable in connecting with colleagues in general. In utilizing the SOAR methodology for strategic planning there is golden opportunity to involve all employees to participate. When using the traditional SWOT tool, there would naturally be apprehension in bringing colleagues into a meeting room that is focusing 50% on their organization's weaknesses. This would naturally link to leadership, discussing threats by competitors may highlight advantages and attract existing employees. Involving colleagues in the goal planning process is a new leadership thought principle. Colleagues are one of the most important stakeholders; it is the colleagues that will make the directive vision of the organization a reality. Involving colleagues in goal setting may sound like a daunting task, but in actuality is very doable.

The SOAR strategic planning process aligns well with Chapter Eight, where we discuss the payoffs from discovering, valuing, and appreciating employee strengths. The same principles of valuing people and focusing on strengths apply in this method of strategic planning for an organization as it does for individuals. Leaders desire for our employees to SOAR, so our organizations will SOAR. Aligning these valuable strengths in the minds, bodies, and souls of the people doing the work propels the organization to greater success and significance. The core of the organization is its colleagues. The organization that connects to the strength of each colleague will create momentum that builds positive influence and excellence.

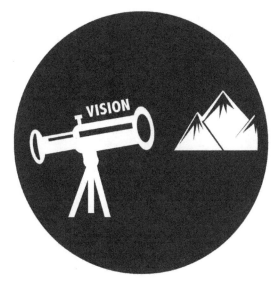

Figure 1

Our Vision Symbol

A telescope trained on a distant mountain is a way to depict vision. This vision symbol reminds us that seeing the destination requires the right altitude and latitude, with the knowledge of where to focus in order to see our destination. The more clearly each colleague in your organization visualizes the arrival point, the more effectively and confidently they can work to propel the organization to reaching that place. It allows them to be aware of the milestones when they see the team moving closer to the vision fruition. It gives hope that the place the organization aspires to reach is attainable.

Any time a colleague sees the vision – like looking through the telescope to see the destination in the distance – it improves their ability to make good decisions and apply their efforts and strengths to the right areas. The main reason for creating the Corporate Transcendence™ Vision Symbol[iv] (along with the eight remaining Corporate Transcendence™ Value Symbols discussed and illustrated throughout this book) is to provide a visual communication symbol that can be used to recognize and reward colleagues at any level when their actions and attitudes convey and support the organization's foundational principles. Leaders play a critical role in crafting the vision, but bringing the vision into reality rests in the hands of the men and women who complete the daily healthcare tasks.

CULTURE TRANSFORMATION ACTION STEPS:

FRONTLINE STAFF:

Do you know what your organization's vision statement says? Is it posted on a wall or in a place where you could easily find it? The vision represents a future desired state of being that will directly affect all colleagues. Take a moment to reflect on how the vision statement relates to your performance as a direct caregiver or frontline support. The realized success will be based largely on the sensitivity, awareness, and focus you give to the organization's vision. Open your mind to be actively engaged and empowered to support the future desired and make a positive difference in people's lives and the organization's success.

MANAGERIAL LEADERSHIP:

Recognize your role in leading by empowering frontline colleagues in supporting and ultimately achieving the vision. It is the daily consistency and persistent efforts of management and frontline colleagues that find effective ways to fulfill the vision. Creating inter-departmental teams to solve problems and gain feedback from staff can strengthen your strategies for achieving the vision in very real ways. Do not forget to celebrate what is valued.

EXECUTIVE LEADERSHIP:

At the executive level, it is our responsibility to find a vision expansive enough to energize and sustain continual growth for the organization. Vision is what sustains colleagues when the unexpected happens; so view and engage problems in light of the vision, and help your team stay in touch with it. This will solidify your organizational identity and fuel momentum toward the vision. Vision is a future destination point that must be traveled daily.

CHAPTER 5

Leadership Environment: Marks the Journey

• • •

*"The growth and development of people is
the highest calling of a leader."*

JOHN C. MAXWELL

DEFINING LEADERSHIP

In a healthy way, every colleague in the organization should be thought of as a leader. Colleagues influence one another and lead their work – and themselves – each day. Leadership is both a natural personal attribute and also a skill which can be developed. To be an effective leader you have to cultivate the ability to take people with you toward a goal or a vision. The magic of leadership is the ability to cast a vision and inspire people to join with you in order to achieve it. Leadership is about partnering, not how many followers tag behind you. Titles, position, and rank do not make a leader. But if a leader's words and behavior earns the trust of others so that they align and respect that person, then they are a leader. Leaders often cast vision based on faith. They see something that is not tangible or realized, but they believe strong enough to develop something that is nonexistent.

A Culture of Collaboration

To build a culture that heals instead of a culture that kills there must be a philosophy of leadership that embraces teams and collaborators. Collaboration and team leadership has been shown to reduce and prevent events that can be harmful within the organization.

The type of leadership culture created – not the individual leader – will define the future of healthcare. This reality is evidenced by a 10-year, groundbreaking study evaluating the relationship between serious accidents and organizational leadership in the marine industry in Torkel Soma of Propel in Oslo, Norway. What was defined as laissez fare or solo leadership cultures were three to five times more likely to incur a service accident than culture that practice collaboration leadership environment.

Cultures that fostered collaborative leadership encourage shared responsibilities and collaboration across all departments. In laissez faire leadership, failures were seen as critical learning points. The study revealed the likelihood of more serious accidents and mistakes are inversely related to the collaborative and learning maturity of the leadership culture practiced. In practice, collaborative leadership yields fewer mishaps for organizations.

A Center for Creative Leadership (CCL) survey of 500 top executives revealed that one of the top leadership practices most needed and least practiced was cross-functional leadership collaboration. The research concludes most executives understood the importance of collaboration across an organization and that collaborative leadership was critical to outcomes, but it was not found to be embraced in the organizations. There was obvious struggle with leadership's development of this type of collaboration.

Leadership Pit Falls

Healthcare leadership has been dominated by a traditional myopic leadership model. In fact, there has been a lot of effort in the past 30 years to bring healthcare into a business model that will yield higher financial returns for stakeholders and stockholders. Healthcare executives lead their healthcare organizations like other financial successful businesses in America.

Suits in boardrooms have become the norm and leadership seemed to favor a more aristocratic leadership style. This profitability approach has been driven to the point that many healthcare colleagues and providers feel tension between serving mankind and the goals of obtaining large financial returns. This dichotomy of the caregivers and administration's purpose and mission has often led to non-trusting relationships between healthcare executives and healthcare providers. A "we-they" relationship mentality develops.

Disappointingly, during my career in various venues, I have heard statements like, "the powers that be, only care about the bottom line – not the patients." In fact, a medical resident student explained to me that in his medical school residences, the students were advised by respected mentors to never trust the hospital or healthcare administration in their future career. Unfortunately, I have often heard this message from providers and colleagues through the years and it is a culprit to a collaborative team model. Personal expressions similar or like this are unfortunate but clearly demonstrate the divisive leadership model that has been steeped traditionally in healthcare.

This may not always be the case, but Healthcare leaders of the future must consider how they lead, and grasp the understanding of how their leadership style affects the organizational culture. Relationship-building is the single most important leadership characteristic for a healthcare leader to possess today. This is due to the necessity for leadership to understand that collaborative and team leadership will be required to meet the demands of healthcare reform.

Collaborative team leadership will be necessary for fluid employee communication, high colleague engagement, and empowerment. With collaborative team leadership an organization can transcend the traditional model, creating a culture that heals instead of a culture that kills. The days of "do as I say because I say so" are over. Leaders must develop and foster cultures of excellence through building relationships and shared collaborative team leadership. Leadership that connects in this way produces an empowering work environment, and encourages everyone to have input, be accountable and do their best in all situations.

Healthy Culture

Organizational culture matters. The healthiest cultures will be the driving force behind the most successful future healthcare organization. Healthcare will win the day when its leaders think in terms of cross-functional team leadership and develop organizational infrastructure to support and sustain it.

Cultures need to be learning environments that foster and sustain open and learning communication that is free to question and explore the existing healthcare environment. A leadership culture that is marked by closed communication and led with fear, intimidation, and negative consequences for employees is a failing culture. This type of, status quo environment needs to die and be reborn with new cultural norms. Open, honest communication and authentic transparency should be the default always if we are to deliver the quality of care people deserve.

To reap full benefits of collaborative leadership, this leadership behavior must be embedded as part of the organization's culture and not be confined to a few select leaders. It must flow in a 360° manner within the organization. The leadership culture affects everything, because it touches everything. Healthcare financial daily operations, quality of care, employee satisfaction, and patient satisfaction are directly impacted by the leadership that is modeled and resulting culture of the organization.

Getting the culture "right" in healthcare has become a mandate and not an option. Today with value-based purchasing, mediocre care is no longer acceptable. Financial rewards are tied to patient clinical outcomes. So the question becomes, "how will twenty-first century healthcare leaders embrace this brave new world?" This new healthcare world is drastically different from traditional leadership. Now we must lead with our eyes on the patients' needs in a holistic manner to deliver the patient quality outcomes that are linked to reimbursements.

Twenty first century leadership begins with establishing the "right" culture. Delivering value-based medicine in a traditional healthcare culture is like trying to force an elephant through the eye of a needle. Organizations that fail to prepare the culture to deliver the new era of care will result in an inability to deliver the quality of care expected and could ultimately destroy the organization.

HEALTHCARE CORNERSTONES
Leading a healthcare organization requires effective, intentional focus on the Four Cornerstones of Healthcare. If we – as leaders – want to transform our unhealthy organization into a healthy, healing one, these four areas must have our attention. These four cornerstones are Culture (work environment), Quality (patient care and experience), Finance (profitability), and Governance (regulatory compliance). These cornerstones create the internal structure that maintains healthcare. Each is interdependent to a large degree on each other. As a leader, these cornerstones are your main drive and priority.

THE CORNERSTONE OF CULTURE
If you ask many healthcare leaders how much time they designate to culture development in their organization, the answer may surprise you. Often, time spent by leadership on culture assessment, cultivation, and development falls at a low percent. Traditional healthcare did not make organizational culture a topic of discussion or a priority. Cultural transformation was not recognized as something needed.

Historically, healthcare administration education has not addressed it as an important part of leadership's work. There seems to be an assumption that culture takes care of itself. In this mindset lies a major misconception. Traditional healthcare culture model has been mainly top-down. Often, culture even became more anarchical – a culture of "us" against "them." The "us" consisted of the providers and employees; "them" takes the form of administration. Leadership and management seem to have their own closed club, or ivory tower. This culture formed a great divide. When there was communication between "us" and "them, it was a monologue of goals and objectives that one or the other party wanted to accomplish. Trust is an issue in the "us/them" world. Decisions are made in silos and others below the upper circle were rarely asked for input.

Serving as a leader in a traditional healthcare culture in the past years, I now know firsthand some of the leadership gaps faced. Minimal discussion took place in regard to the type of culture we wanted to create by senior leadership or board members. In fact, cultural discussions were not part of the agendas or on the table. Values were sometimes listed within the mission and vision statements, but not discussed beyond that. We talked about our employees and work environment when we needed to fix a problem like patient dissatisfaction or low employee morale. We did not address culture in a systemic way. The topic on culture seemed to be an add-on of less value and not a priority. It was just not that important with so many other competing needs.

If you asked healthcare leaders how much time they feel they have to spend on culture development they may say "little" to "none." As I reflect on my early years as a senior leader, I realize that we mostly extinguishing fires to the point that we were not aware of the answer inside our walls as part of a sustainable solution to extinguish fires. Many hours were focused on how to fix people instead of how to utilize people to help us lead the organization more effectively. The answer to healthcare excellence was right under our nose, right in the room. As leaders we were not able then to make a connection that sustainable excellence grows from the inside out.

Barriers to Healthcare Culture Transformation

The barrier to addressing culture in a systemic approach by healthcare leaders has to do with a number of factors. For example, some healthcare leaders do not embrace that cultural transformation is an ongoing process and is needed for an organization to achieve and maintain excellence. This is a prevalent mindset in the fee-for-service healthcare environment. Other leaders have expressed that it takes too much time and energy to focus on culture development. They feel their plates are overflowing and do not have time or energy to work on a culture transformation infrastructure or plan. Even more critically, a leader may feel they do not have the skills and training to be successful in implementation of a cultural transformation initiative that would be sustainable.

Today, more than ever, the spot light is focused on the value and power that a positive organizational culture delivers. As our healthcare institution leaders become aware of the need for culture transformation, we see the increasing need for leadership to cast a vision for culture development and to provide the training and support for all colleagues to help create that culture.

Culture Cultivation Is Far From Easy

Culture development and transformation is not a microwave process. It takes initiatives on multiple levels and constant leading and oversight for a new culture to take root and grow. There are few leaders in healthcare who possess cultural development expertise. Leaders cannot possibly be all things to all people. Well-meaning leaders often settle for a motivational speaker that comes and goes in a few hours, or a flavor-of-the-month training in how to be nice to our customers. Neither delivers the lasting effect that is needed to transform and sustain the work environment to one of continuous excellence. A systemic corporate wide solution is required.

THE CORNERSTONE OF QUALITY

In the healthcare industry, quality of care is essential. Consumers want a healthcare provider they feel will take the best care of them, effectively addressing their health concerns. There are many questions of why there are so many poor health outcome ratings among Americans, compared to other financially influential countries. In a 2014 report by The Commonwealth Fund, The United States health system was ranked 11th out of 11 of the world's most industrialized countries. The United States ranked first in healthcare expenditure per capita. The 10 best performing healthcare systems were France, Italy, San Marino, Andorra, Malta, Singapore, Spain, Oman, Austria, and Japan. Our ranking places us behind those of Norway, Portugal, Monaco, Greece, Iceland, Luxembourg, Netherlands, United Kingdom, Ireland, Switzerland, Belgium, Colombia, Sweden, Cyprus, Germany, Saudi Arabia, United Arab Emirates, Israel, Morocco, Canada, Finland, Australia, Chile, Denmark, Dominica, and Costa Rica. Unfortunately concerns among the public and stakeholders have not diminished, but grown. America remains the highest in cost for healthcare and has some of the worst patient outcomes.[v]

A complex problem of this magnitude needs a systemic, sustainable solution to transform America's healthcare. It must begin with how we operate day-to-day; it must begin with culture transformation from the traditional practice of healthcare. Culture has to be front and center in the board rooms, because it has too long been the elephant in the room.

BEST PRACTICES

Americans and all healthcare payers want to know that when a patient is seen, the organization has taken the necessary steps to ensure the best possible outcomes for the patient. Best practices and evidence-based care should be delivered using proven protocols and procedures. Excellent organizations are expected to be hardwired for quality, and continuous improvement. Quality accrediting organizations such as The Joint Commission have focused on campaigns in healthcare to encourage excellence in specific areas, and have safety goals established for best practices in hand washing, medication reconciliation, patient identification, improved communication among caregivers, reducing the risk of healthcare-associated infections, and many other focused areas.

Focus on the cornerstone of quality, has resulted in the many standards of care published by The Joint Commission. The Joint Commission is the largest accrediting body for the healthcare industry. These standards represent minimal standards needed in providing quality of care. The Joint Commission encourages organizations to continuously improve and to always seek to exceed these standards and create best practices.[vi]

Performance Improvement and Innovation

Continuous quality and performance improvement is vital to the culture and health of an organization. A high reliability organization understands that there are always learning opportunities for improving a process, and there is value in being proactive in preventing potential risk or addressing mistakes when they occur. Today in many instances in healthcare, leaders search for a fast and furious fix to improve operations. One performance improvement model that has been a staple for many organizations, and is supported by The Joint Commission, is "Plan Do Study Act" or PDSA. This process for problem solving has been successful in the market for many years. The PDSA model is a tool for performance improvement widely used in healthcare today.

The PDSA acronym stands for:

PLAN: Plan a change or a test, aimed at improvement.

DO: Carry out the change or test, preferably in a small scale.

STUDY: Study the results. What did we learn? What went wrong?

ACT: Adopt the change, abandon it, or run through the cycle again.

The PDSA tool has served many organizations well, but I would like to suggest you consider innovating and customizing your own process improving acronym so that it reflects your culture. When your process improvement system reflects your culture, colleagues become more engaged and have more ownership of the process improvement tool. The two should be intertwined to the point that they are indistinguishable.

For example, colleagues at a large North Carolina community healthcare system (CommWell Health[vii]) decided their culture transformation program would be named Eagle Excellence. In keeping with the Eagle Excellence mindset, the colleagues created a substitution for PDSA, using the acronym TALONS. TALONS, being the claws of an eagle, reminded them of their desire to achieve Eagle Excellence everyday as they dig their claws into operational improvements in culture, quality, finance, and governance. The TALONS acronym represents the following elements:

TEAM: Who needs to be involved? Include colleagues across disciplines. Remember nothing happens in a vacuum.

ACKNOWLEDGE: Acknowledge the problem. Define the Opportunity. What are we trying to improve? Who are the stakeholders?

LEARN: Understand the current situation. Map the current processes and provide data to measure current performance. Study the cause. Brainstorm the possible reasons why the opportunity needs improvement. Determine the root cause of the problem.

OPERATIONALIZE: Describe the improvement you are going to work on. Develop an implementation strategy.

NOTE: How successful was the implementation? Review data to measure performance.

SUSTAIN: How are we going to standardize the process? When is the next cycle of improvement for this process?

A nice crosswalk is seen between the PDSA and TALONS model. Literally the sky is the limit when colleagues brainstorm, and the end result is brilliant in my experience.

LEAN SIX SIGMA

Another popular tool that has been the default for healthcare organizations for many years is referred to as LEAN Six Sigma. This workflow process tool has been in the market since early 1900's originating in the Toyota automotive industry. LEAN has succeeded in healthcare by focusing on value creation for the end customer with minimal waste as performance in processes is improved. While LEAN Six Sigma has many positive attributes to outline workflow, I caution that improving workflow processes only will not provide the cure for all that needs to improve in healthcare today.[viii]

MALCOLM BALDRIGE WORKFLOW

Stated in the Malcolm Baldrige Criteria for Performance Excellence, all key processes need to have clear and concise steps that outline workflows. These criteria ask how your organization designs, manages, and improves its healthcare services and work processes, and how it improves operational effectiveness to deliver value to patents and other customers, and to achieve organizational sustainability. Each criterion illustrates the importance of workflow processes mapped out in all areas of an organization, with a high reliable culture to support and sustain it. Note the words "high reliable culture" in the previous sentence. For example, it is difficult for a group of individuals to develop optimal workflow processes, if they have not been trained on successful team dynamics. This is why a culture that supports colleague's personal and professional development is critical to performance improvement and workflow design.[ix]

The Author Solution

Recently entering the United States from Scotland is an instinctual and knowledge-driven process-mapping software called "Author." This product is being distributed by Corporate Memory Solutions (CMS). Corporate Memory Solutions offers business process mapping solutions (workflow design) and utilizes highly engaged colleagues to create a systemic memory and operational efficiency that becomes part of the overall daily corporate memory. CMS understands that improving processes and hardwiring memory for organizational efficiencies and effectiveness is needed for all areas of the organization such as finance, culture, quality, and governance, to deliver a high reliability organization. Corporate Memories Solutions also advocates that healthcare organizations that have invested in culture development are most successful and sustainable for ongoing process improvement for their organization. Culture development of excellence is priority and marries their concept of mapping to the culture development process itself.[x]

Reimbursing Based on Patient Experience

The government has also begun to use patient clinical outcome measures that are tied to reimbursement to encourage improved health outcomes. The Medicare Hospital Consumer Assessment of Healthcare Providers and Systems (HCAHPS[xi]) survey also asks patients about the quality of healthcare patient experience. The better the patient experience, the more monetary reward the healthcare entity receives. The importance of the patient's experience has resulted in an interesting phenomenon: the title of Chief Patient Experience Officer (CPEO). There has been a significant rise in the CPEO title in the United States. Some organizations have recognized the pivotal element of patient experience as part of quality by recruiting business experts like the Ritz Carlton to improve their ability to serve healthcare consumers in a first class way. Unfortunately, a link between this strategy and improvement of clinical outcomes for the patient can be a challenge.

CLINICAL OUTCOMES AND THE AFFORDABLE CARE ACT

More focus on quality in healthcare has been legislated through the Patient Protection and Affordable Care Act.[xii] Accountable Care Organizations bring to the table value-based cost sharing programs like the one being used for Medicare patients.[xiii] There are over 30 patient clinical outcomes being monitored for Medicare patients that chose to enroll. This will relate to saving the government considerable money if obtained through better healthcare management such as seen in the Patient-Centric Model of care.

The National Quality Strategy Mandated under ACA released March 21, 2011 was built on a Triple Aim Strategy.[xiv] The first aim is for better care; the desire is to improve the overall quality of care by making healthcare more patient-centered, reliable, accessible, and safe. The second aim is for improved access to care; the desire is to improve the health of the United States population by supporting proven interventions to address behavioral, social, and environmental determinants of health to deliver higher quality care. The third aim is to deliver affordable care; the desire is to reduce the cost of quality healthcare for individuals, families, employers, and government.[xv] If there was a fourth aim decided to be added in the future, I would suggest that it would be this: create a culture of excellence within healthcare organizations through healthcare colleagues or workforce.

THE CORNERSTONE OF FINANCE

As of 2014, healthcare in the United States represents 17.1% of the Gross National Product (GNP).[xvi] This represents 3 trillion dollars, or $9,523 per person. This includes public and private health expenditures, covering health services both preventative and curative, family planning, nutritional activities, and emergency aid.[xvii]

A FEE-FOR-SERVICE WORLD

Historically, healthcare in America has been a fee-for-service industry, which means a service is provided and a fee is charged and paid.

Fee-for-service is the typical American way of economic reimbursement. Retail industries operate this way, stimulating the marketplace in the development of new pharmaceuticals, technology, and equipment to be used to support the patient in the healthcare industry. The manufacturers are financially rewarded when the healthcare industry utilizes their product, and we in healthcare pass the cost on to the federal and state healthcare plans, as well as, to third party commercial payers or the consumer. Overutilization of services became costly in diagnostic equipment, special types of surgeries and treatment for fatal diseases, and more. Patients not on a government health plan such a Medicare or Medicaid or who have medical insurance from a commercial entity fall into the population of people who chose not to be insured or cannot afford healthcare insurance. Cost to people with insurance or who can afford to pay for healthcare has been high and, in many cases, their premiums helped to cover cost for healthcare organizations serving those who could not or would not pay for care. Government disproportionate share programs for indigent care also helped to offset the cost of caring for those uninsured, using annual reimbursement back to healthcare organizations. Quality is always expected for a service rendered, but was not a significant factor in the reimbursement formula for healthcare in the past. Reimbursement had more to do with the overhead cost of doing business than the patient clinical outcome and the overall health of the patient.

THE IMPACT OF CULTURE ON FINANCES

Finance is a key Cornerstone in healthcare because it influences everything in regard to the delivery of care. This is not a book on healthcare finance, but the importance of creating a healthy organizational culture that will always improve the bottom line. In fact, we experience compounding financial benefits - by being the employer of choice by attracting great caregivers and talented providers, and becoming the provider of choice for patients. The financial picture will also improve when we garner value-based reimbursement from improved patient care experience, and patient health outcomes. The return on investment (ROI) is measurable by the above factors and others, when we invest in the people and the culture. Culture is a significant part of the financial landscape for organizations.

A Case Study in Financial Turnaround

The claims and principles in the book are not just a manifestation of my hopes for healthcare; they are also realities that have been achieved in the past six years within a healthcare system. My work was with a large community healthcare system in the role of turnaround CEO. It was stated empathetically by a Joint Commission surveyor who evaluated us just 10 months into my new role: "This organization had been burned to the ground. You must be living in hell."

At the time, I was brought in to lead the efforts in saving the organization, the debt load was upwards of $8 million and bankruptcy was looming on the horizon. Not only was the organization unable to make payroll, and accounts payable months past due, the accounts receivable was over $3 million with no hope of collecting due to operational dysfunctions. Every state and federal grant – representing approximately 50% of the budget – was in jeopardy. Due to precipitous loss of staff through voluntary and involuntary terminations, layoffs, and a deadly sick culture, there was little left to turn the organization.

The journey began with a deathly ill healthcare organization, but through the relentless efforts of the incredible people, the organization was transformed into a thriving healthcare system. Drastic changes with rebuilt departments from the ground up, created an award-winning organization, with the vision to become a premier organization in the nation.

It has been six years from the beginning of the transformation process. The organization has gone from over $8 million in debt to under

$1.4 million in long term debt. In that time, the organization has received 36 National Service Excellence awards. Patient satisfaction scores are consistently high, with many over 90% across all departments and office locations throughout multiple counties. Financial indicators are all above bank and healthcare industry standards and benchmarks. Employee and provider satisfaction is high and represented by high retention and low turnover.

Successful Joint Commission accreditation for Ambulatory and Behavioral Health and Primary Care Medical Home, to recognition of programs by the Health Resources and Service Administration (HRSA) Ryan White as best practice based on high risk populations for patient quality outcomes. The organization has risen quickly through applying the principles and practices explained in this book. Leaders can cement the cornerstone of finance by aggressively developing the culture and people in their organization.

THE CORNERSTONE OF GOVERNANCE

How much governance is required to ensure best care possible in healthcare today? The answer today to that question has grown to a mammoth amount. It seems everyone has a stake in the regulation and governance of healthcare. From the governing board of directors, municipal, county, and state ordinances, state federal agencies that influence reimbursement such as for Centers for Medicare & Medicaid Services (CMS), the Center for Disease Control (CDC), Health Resources and Services Administration (HRSA), legislative acts affecting healthcare operations from malpractice to the Patient Protection and Affordable Care Act (ACA), the Health Insurance Portability and Accountability Act (HIPAA), Corporate Compliance, Office of Inspector General (OIG), healthcare grantors – the list continues. All told, these entities issue hundreds of thousands of regulations for healthcare organizations to adhere to.

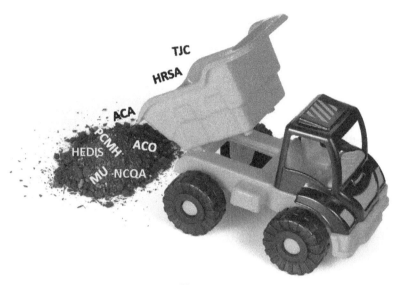

Figure 2

Dump Truck Syndrome (DTS)

When it comes to the governance cornerstone, organizations are dealing with massive overload. Large dump trucks are needed to haul around all of the requirements and mandates the healthcare industry is forced to comply to. With so many entities providing oversight, the task seems almost impossible. Healthcare workers travel to conferences to learn more about what is the new or latest information in the dump truck to bring home. Too often the governance "dump truck" backs up to the healthcare colleagues, and buries them once again in more regulations and advisory statements. The Dump Truck delivers lots of "must do's," providing little in the way of strategy for how to comply.

The reason there is such a drain on our energy coming from the governance sector is because our culture has not been designed or developed to support it. Without the correct culture design, the reaction becomes an obsession to check off compliance boxes. Anyone who misses a check box ends up becoming a scapegoat, blamed for failing to meet the demands of governance guidelines and regulation. Everyone gets beat up under this model. It polarizes and isolates departments as they try to shore up their defensive strategies and not end up losing in the blame game.

In this type of culture, often one department is succeeding while another fails; this indicates that organization have become siloes, creating subcultures in order to survive. Poor performance will come from the departments who have sicker subcultures. When a department performs poorly, it is people who are blamed. Unfortunately, most often it is not actually the PEOPLE in the department, it is the fact that the people in one culture are in an environment that supports them less. People cannot carry the demands of governance if they already have the weight of a sick culture on their backs every day.

Demands of Government through Culture Development

The treatment for "Dump Truck Syndrome" is healing the culture. We cannot improve our performance in meeting governance until we get the culture in shape. Culture is the sticky stuff that makes it possible for our organization to evolve and stretch to meet the demands of what is in the dump truck. Until there is a healthy culture, organizations cannot be hardwired to consistently produce and meet the enormous demands of governance. Incredible things happen when organizations develop an ownership culture where people are empowered to work in and develop their strengths. When organizations have this, staff can take on elements of governance and create methods and strategies that work to implement and meet its demands. Equipping and empowering people will result in them discovering, and bringing back solutions to the organization to meet the demands of governance that are more manageable for everyone.

Start With the Culture

Let's keep this simple. Culture is the first cornerstone leadership must address. Continually developing the culture should be a major ongoing leadership goal. In fact, to create a workplace of excellence that is strong financially, has great patient quality outcomes, and meets all government regulatory requirements, the Culture Cornerstone must be leadership's number one priority. Knowing where to best spend your energy can be the most difficult part as a leader. As Stephen Covey said, "The main thing is to keep the main thing the main thing." But how do you do that when it seems every area of the organization needs attention?

The Tripp 3-3-3-1 Leadership Principle
Structure for Time Effectiveness

Culture	30%
Quality	30%
Finance	30%
Governance	10%

CORPORATE
TRANSCENDENCE

Figure 3

THE 3-3-3-1 LEADERSHIP PRINCIPLE

I have developed what I call "The 3-3-3-1 Leadership Principle." As a CEO, 30% of my time is spent on culture development and improvements, 30% to quality of care improvement, 30% to financial efficacy, and 10% to governance. Most healthcare leaders spend the majority of their time on finance and governance, then quality and culture gets the leftover attention. The 3-3-3-1 Leadership Principle will, for many, be a complete flip in the leadership paradigm. Leaders who lead by spending 30% of their energy and time focusing on culture, quality, and financial elements FIRST, will find that governance will only require 10% of their time.

Governance represents all regulatory standards and compliance and is full of mandates as discussed earlier as DTS. That does not change the priority focus by leadership on the cornerstone of culture. Remember that the Culture cornerstone is like the mortar that stabilizes Quality, Finance, and Governance and keeps them in place. In other words if you are struggling in Quality, Finance, and Governance, then concentrate on improving the culture. Culture is people and without their engagement and support the healthcare organization is a shell of brick and mortar.

People are the breath, life, pulse of the organization; when they succeed, the organization succeeds. To lead an organization that represents excellence, transcendence, and is distinguished from other healthcare organizations is a result of intentionally improving organizational culture on an infinite basis. Leaders will obtain an amazing return for investing in their people and this investment in return will drive all areas of the organization. Leaders and colleagues want the best healthcare professionals in the industry breaking down doors to work for them. Colleagues that remain long term will build many ladders of greatness for the future within the organization.

LEADERSHIP CORE VALUES

Leadership core values are vital, but rarely seem to be discussed when evaluating leaders for job opportunities. The job description represents responsibilities around a specific scope of work, but it does not describe or reveal how it will be carried out in reality. How will a leader's core values play into what is expected of them from their job description?

Abraham Lincoln was an individual whose core values powerfully influenced his leadership behavior. He valued human life and the belief that man should be free. His values influenced his leadership as President. It stands to reason; if he had not possessed these personal core values, history could have been written very differently. Lincoln's core values drastically changed and influenced the lives of many future generations. Leadership core values matter. To better understand an individual leader, it is necessary to look deeper into the makeup or traits of the individual leader. Leaders, like people have beliefs and values that have been developed and instilled in them from a young age.

A Leader's core values and their personal core values will naturally align. Much time is spent on examining the needed employee's characteristics for an organization to be successful. But first and foremost we must look at the character of its leaders. This will directly dictate the organizational culture of the organization as well as its future success.

LEADERSHIP CONNECTION
Leadership is a vital piece of any culture of excellence. There must be positive leadership characteristics to align with building the organization's core of excellence.

The bestselling author and my long time mentor, John C. Maxwell defines leadership as influence; nothing more and nothing less. The more I have studied this concept, the more I agree. Having a title of leader or Chief Executive Officer or President does not define the leader's ability, only the position held. Leaders define themselves by the impact they have on others in achieving the strategic vision of the organization. In his book *Leadership Gold,* John Maxwell states that if you are a leader and cross the finish line alone that is a sign of poor leadership. A leader will bring all his followers alongside him across the finish line to reach their goals together.

Dan Cathy, the President of Chick-Fil-A, shared at a John Maxwell training conference that the CEO title in his company was defined as the Chief Encouragement Officer and the COO as the Chief Opportunity Officer. What a wonderful way a leader can demonstrate their desire to build a personal relationship with all colleagues. As a CEO, I adopted the title of Chief Encouragement Officer and it made a wonderful difference with my colleagues. Some leadership management titles can be perceived as separating employees to levels of superiority and inferiority and create silos and diminish team spirit. Leaders must make intentional efforts to stay connected to their employees. If a colleague was employed by a Chief

Encouragement Officer versus a Chief Executive Officer there may be a feeling of sharing a more common ground to build a relationship upon. People like to associate with encouraging people.

A Chief Encouragement Officer title sends a message by the leader as one that values the colleagues and their work. There is a sense of empathy transferred to the colleagues that the leader feels what it is like to walk in their shoes.

Leadership influence is essential in creating and developing an organization of excellence. To establish the infrastructure it must be accomplished with a culture of empathy, overarching vision, understanding personal strengths, momentum, valuing individual significance, equipping and empowerment and the right leadership core values. These vital organization characteristics are the initial foundational principles to prepare an organization for excellence.

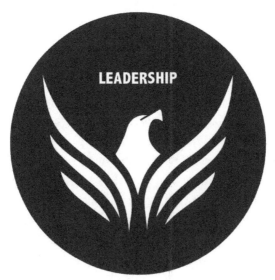

Figure 4

OUR LEADERSHIP SYMBOL

The majestic Eagle was chosen to symbolize the attributes of Leadership. It may be given to anyone regardless of their position, title, job description, or responsibilities in the organization. The Corporate Transcendence™ Leadership Symbol[xix] represents a colleague behavior of stepping up in work experiences, building collaboration, and the support of all the leadership values within the organization. The Eagle is a reminder to all colleagues that they can soar, rise above, and lead regardless of any situation in the organization and beyond.

Culture Transformation Action Steps:

Frontline Staff:

Leadership on the front line begins with how well you lead yourself. Being committed to your best performance and being comfortable with your work accountability. Model collaborative team leadership, so your colleagues will learn to trust and rely on you. As a frontline leader, value yourself and others by looking for opportunities to enhance your knowledge and skills, so you can enhance the contributions you give your team.

Managerial Leadership:

Initiate and establish a relationship that lives by trust and transparency between yourself and direct reports. Recognize that frontline colleagues are incredibly valuable in brainstorming solutions and innovating to improve and build efficiency in workflows. Your leadership effectiveness will be based on the quality of your relationship with your colleagues. Demonstrate that you value their perspective and expertise. Celebrate the value of the accomplishments by individuals and teams. Invite colleagues to step up in more formal leadership roles by leading a team or helping lead department meetings or having a part of the agenda. Charge them with problem solving and critical thinking to come up with innovative solutions to continuously improve the work environment.

Executive Leadership:

Expanded responsibility and authority comes hand-in-hand with accepting a higher degree of accountability. You will foster leadership by promoting an atmosphere of valuing and giving colleagues space to express their opinions. Be willing to initiate and maintain transparency. Learn to bring your strengths to the table with the mindset of complementing – rather than competing with – the strengths of others. Dig for a high-level decision-making and problem-solving environment. Make sure that the executive leadership is focused on Organizational Culture and HEALTH, and reaching its vision in a way that continuously develops, values, and places people at all levels in their top position of strengths. Stay closely connected to the middle management and frontline colleagues to cultivate relationships.

CHAPTER 6

Empathy: Humanity's Need

• • •

*"You never really understand a person until you
consider things from his point of view. Until you
climb into his skin and walk around in it."*

ATTICUS FINCH

DEFINING EMPATHY

Empathy is deeply valuing other people and developing understanding of
what others are feeling through shared experience. To be truly empathetic,
you have to raise your awareness of the emotions and needs of those around
you, and put yourself into their shoes. Empathy goes beyond the caregiver-
to-patient relationship. Colleague-to-colleague empathy is crucial. Empathy
among colleagues requires recognizing the commonalities that transcend
the uniqueness of our departments and roles. When people come to work,
they bring their own high and lows of life with them. Empathetic colleagues
coming in touch with those high and lows as needed. Challenges in day-to-
day life in general is part of everyone's life. You do not have to meddle in
people's personal lives in order to be empathetic.

Identifying with any shared feelings due to our similar experience in
that situation prepares us to extend compassion, caring, and kindness to
them. Empathy requires retaining sensitivity to the humanity of people.
It is very easy to become desensitized to people and their day-to-day

struggles, but by choosing to value people and reach out to them on a human level, we create an environment of empathy, where patients and colleagues feel valued and can thrive. Keeping our radar trained on others' feelings allows colleagues to enjoy the highs of celebrating happy events in their colleagues' lives, and shortens our reaction time when a tragedy occurs. Caring behavior demonstrates empathy.

My Empathy Experience: Trying on Other Shoes

There I was; the Vice President of a community hospital standing in a borrowed uniform from the environmental services department. It was dull and dingy and I felt dreary just wearing it. My mentor for the day, "James," didn't seem to mind his attire. I followed him for a full 9-hour shift while taking mental notes of improvements that could be made to assist James in his job, and create efficiencies for the unit. I had a task list, and was ready to "make things happen." During our 30-minute lunch I was reminded of the reason I decided to shadow employees like James. He shared with me about the struggles he faced completing certain jobs, and the sadness he carried daily thinking about his sick child. He expressed the guilt of making overtime to meet work demands to help support his family versus spending time with them.

The light bulb went off as my focus shifted and I remembered that shadowing employees wasn't just about systems, but was about building relationships. I wanted to build trust. I wanted to truly understand their daily struggles on a level where I was able to experience it myself. I wanted to know their hearts, why they did the work they did, and what motivated them. I wanted to get inside their thoughts and their hearts. I needed to walk in their shoes to accomplish this.

I continued the practice of shadowing employees in different departments over the next seven months, squeezing this time into my already overbooked schedule. As the word got out among frontline staff that I was working alongside employees, I began to receive request from employees requesting me to work with them when I was scheduled for their department. The purpose of the request I learned was that as a senior leader, they desired for me to see firsthand how hard they worked and so I could appreciate their daily efforts, whether it was drawing blood or washing large pots. The employees wanted my admiration for their efforts and to feel valued by leadership as well as other colleagues. Upon reflection, I began to realize there was a viable lesson to be learned in their request.

I wore no fashionable business suit, no genuine leather heels, no important nametag screaming to the employees that I was one of the C-Suite people in the organization. I traded all this in for hair nets, scrubs, and burgundy over-washed polo shirts. Instead of sitting in strategic leadership meetings, or behind my large, wooden desk I worked alongside employees pushing carts, mopping floors, serving food, drawing blood, and throwing out trash. In my journey of learning, I felt my heart started to beat more like theirs. My thoughts seemed to align with theirs, and my feet ached like theirs after a long day of manual labor.

I realized how drab and gloomy I felt wearing the uniforms provided to our housekeeping staff. I realized that more fashionable, colorful uniform for the housekeeping staff instead of dark burgundy ones could make a difference in how a person felt about herself. A uniform may appear to be a small thing, but it can make a big difference. More importantly, I gained such valuable insight about what it actually meant to be a non-management employee in the hospital I help lead. Learning so much about their daily challenges and struggles, my empathy for their efforts measurably increased. Understanding them on a whole new level created a new awareness on the inside and a burning desire to advocate for their needs more aggressively than I had ever before.

THE POWER OF EMPATHY IN BUSINESS

Empathy can transform leaders into powerful change agents, but it can also transform the business itself. In a recent study of more than 600 companies, results showed that those companies who focused on organizational health and understood their employees yielded twice as much financial performance as those who did not.[xx] Although finding time to shadow employees or learn about their struggles in a hands-on way may be a big challenge, research is pointing to the fact that companies cannot afford NOT to be intentional about developing relationships that lead to a deep understanding of employee needs and desires. This is certainly what I have found to be true in my research and work experiences.

More than just understanding, leaders must make empathy a core value of their leadership practice. A culture of empathy must be palpable and supported from the Chief Encouragement Office (CEO), the C-Suite, middle management, and frontline staff. Initiatives with daily practices have to be hardwired into the infrastructure to create, develop, and build this culture trait of empathy. For me, gaining an even deeper empathy required me to shadow my employees to literally "put myself in their shoes."

If a healthcare leader does not possess the competency of interpersonal relationships including the value of empathy, they will have major problems in a people industry like healthcare. Healthcare is an industry that functions for people and by people. Basing your environment on the value of empathy builds connectivity between all levels, all position titles, and all job descriptions. This connection between employee and employer results in measurable organizational success.

EMPATHY DEFICIT DISORDER

Based on his research and studies in behavioral health, Dr. Douglas LaBier, PhD coined the term "Empathy Deficit Disorder" or EDD. Dr. LaBier determined that EDD is a pervasive condition in America, and a greatly overlooked condition. People have a difficult time stepping outside themselves and dialing into what other people are experiencing. This is especially true for those who feel, think, and believe differently from one another. Are you suffering from some degree of EDD? People suffering from EDD are locked inside themselves in an egocentric world. They are desensitized to the people around them.[xxi]

Empathetic people can maintain their own viewpoints, while understanding the person's emotions, conflicts, and aspirations from their map of the world. Master psychologist Carl Rogers wrote "being empathic is a complex, demanding, strong yet subtle and gentle way of being." He simply explained empathy as a special way of coming to know another person, a kind of attuning and understanding. When empathy is extended, it satisfies our needs and wishes for intimacy and rescues us from our feeling of aloneness. He wrote extensively about the necessity of developing the skills of empathy, rather than assuming empathy belong to select personalities.

Empathetic Communication Skills

Empathy is a great communication skill in that a person is sensing the emotions of others. Having empathy allows people to connect and build camaraderie and kindred spirit among each other. A lack of empathy will cause stress or become a barrier to a work relationship. When there is a lack of empathy, many times there is a deficit in communication. This is illustrated in many of the famous Dilbert cartoons that depict an uncaring boss that creates a barrier through the lack of communication and empathy with the employee. This has also been highlighted on the hit TV show "Under Cover Boss."

As fellow workers in healthcare, we need to remember it is not just how we communicate with each other that is important, it is how we connect and empathize with each other that builds trusting relationships and a foundational core for a healthcare environment of excellence.

The mission and motivation of healthcare leaders as an industry is to improve the health and well-being of others in a safe environment. An empathy environment supports this mantra. Practicing organizational mindfulness around empathy helps us to be aware of the perspectives of other people, yet not feel overwhelmed when we encounter people's negative emotions.

EMPATHY REDUCES BULLYING

Studies by Mary Gordon's from the innovative "Roots of Empathy" program found that empathy decreases bullying and aggression among kids and makes them kinder and more inclusive toward their peers. This is based on research that demonstrates we can increase our own level of empathy by actively imagining what someone else may be feeling.[xxii] Empathy is now being taught and encouraged in all grades of schools to reduce bullying among young people.

EMPATHY FIGHTS INEQUALITY

Empathy equips us to identify with one another on a level different than color of skin, ethnicity, gender, religion, age, socioeconomic status and other diverse factors that distinguish humans. True empathy is not a respecter of people; it is genuinely walking in other people's shoes and feeling what they are feeling to the greatest level possible. Having empathy means looking beyond the external to the internal being of a person and finding the common thread as a fellow human beings.

Empathy can be taught, practiced and experienced in many ways in daily activities of life. Understanding and practicing a culture of empathy for healthcare workers will pay it forward to the patients that entrust their healthcare to us. Intentional first steps can be taken by the following three M's:

* Make people feel known.
* Make people feel understood.
* Make people feel they are not alone.

Colleagues are the core of healthcare organizations. What can YOU do or say to show empathy at your workplace? First, you cannot empathize with colleagues that you do not know. I am not talking about taking them to lunch; you can get to know your colleagues in numerous ways. It is not hard to discuss the area they live in, or where they were born, or what they like to do, or why they decided to work with the organization. In fact, you can glean lots of information from just listening. Utilize halls, break, or lunch conversation to get to know your colleagues better. Organizations that invest in personal and professional development also yield many opportunities to foster empathy for colleagues. Being considerate of others feelings is a choice; if developed intentionally, it will become a powerful skill.

Let's think about that for a second. What if your workplace or manager practiced the three "M's" and:

* Made you feel known
* Made you feel understood
* Made you feel like you weren't alone

Empathy has the power to do that. When empathy is a true essential of a workplace culture, people think about others before making decisions.

Employees learn to think about their patients in an empathetic way, for example:

* How would the patient's mother see this situation?
* How would I feel if I were about to get this news today?
* How would I interpret the doctor's message, if it were my spouse in the hospital?

When employees treat each other, and each patient, with empathy; they start seeing, listening, and feeling for another person when they communicate. Their actions show compassion and understanding that make people feel known.

THE HARVARD "MAKING CARING COMMON" PROJECT

The Harvard Graduate School of Education created a project that taught children, parents, caretakers, and community members the skill of empathy in an effort to develop caring, ethical children. The Making Caring

Common project (MCC) is striving to make these values live and breathe in everyday life.[xxiii] The guide offers clear and practical ways to help children become more empathetic.[xxiv]

THIS INCLUDES:

1. Empathizing with your child and model empathy at home.
2. Make caring for others a priority and set positive ethical standards.
3. Provide opportunities for children to practice empathy.
4. Expand your child's circle of concern.

Other words associated with teaching empathy could be nurturing, understanding, love, caring, relating, and communication. What if we took the model above meant for elementary school children and adapted it for our healthcare workplaces? If children can learn the basics of empathy, surely adults can embrace this into our workplace culture.

FOR THE WORKPLACE, ALL EMPLOYEES WOULD BE EXPECTED TO:

1. Empathize with co-workers and reward empathetic behaviors.
2. Make caring for others a priority and set high behavioral standards.
3. Leadership will support and provide opportunities for co-workers to express empathy.
4. Expand employee's circle of concern in the organization.

LEADING EMPATHY

Empathy has been shown scientifically to increase prosocial (helping) behaviors. While American culture has been encouraging individuality rather than empathy, research has uncovered the existence of "mirror neurons" which react to emotions expressed by others and then the brain can reproduce them. This means that when empathy is experienced and felt by another then this behavior is capable of reproducing itself. This is an encouraging discovery. It reminds me of the poem "Everything I Ever Needed to Know I learned in Kindergarten." Children model what is taught them and what they see practiced. Empathy matters in the workplace, our society, nation, and the world.

People create and will sustain the culture in an organization. In other words, it is the colleagues that save the life of a healthcare company, and ultimately the life of the healthcare industry through great leadership. It is important that leadership is in agreement to the fact that people, or the colleagues of healthcare organizations, are its most valuable assets and the source of true transformation in an organization. If you do not believe this statement then it will be hard to grasp the concept of empathy as a major component in developing a culture of excellence.

Empathy cannot exist unless there is an underlying core value of the organization that places others in high regard. This desire is regardless of anything that may distinguish individuals from one another, such as race, gender, ethnicity, socioeconomic status, or religious beliefs. Empathy cannot be a casual conversation, lip service, or a human resources catchphrase. Empathy must be a deeply held, universally agreed-upon value among leadership and within the organization.

When leadership and colleagues are on-board with valuing each individual, then the true work of developing empathy begins. People are at the central work of all that is done in healthcare. Most people would probably agree that caring for people in a healthcare setting creates a unique environment much different from other service industries. A healthcare worker's main role is to care for people experiencing a compromised health condition. These patients are often fearful and suffer from anxiety about their possible or diagnosed health condition. If colleagues are able to truly empathize with each other, then they are most likely to empathize with the patients they care for.

Empathy as a Core Value of Healthcare

Leadership should not underestimate the positive impact active empathy between co-workers could have on their organization. Human beings need to have others to identify with their lives. In fact, I believe our human nature cries out for this. Empathy ties us to our common humanity and protects us from judgment. Judgment often divides us in the workplace. Judgment, in contrast to empathy, works against team participation and team building. Empathy connects us to our intuitive being. When feeling empathy toward another person or being on the receiving end of empathy, it builds a connection between individuals that can craft feelings of trust and acceptance. It is as if a person is able to perceive and understand another person's world. This is important to understand in looking at work processes and flow and the impact it has on teamwork.

Working with this value of empathy is a major building block to the foundation of excellence in healthcare. I am aware that empathy may seem like a simple idea or cliché, but remember the goal is to not just to understand empathy, but to have colleagues model behaviors of empathy toward their colleagues and to the patients they care for on a daily basis. The busy atmosphere of healthcare today may create doubt that a highly empathetic environment could possibly exist. But I assure you; I have led this transformation and know that an empathetic work environment is possible through leadership, value alignment, and personal development of all colleagues.

Empathy as a Practice

Empathy practices must be intentional and start with the leadership of the organization in order for empathy to trickle down the chain of command. If the senior leaders are not displaying empathy, then colleagues will follow their lead. Imagine how a truly empathetic leader could change a workplace. When you are on the receiving end of empathy you may express thankfulness, joy, sadness, or appreciation. Colleagues that I have personally observed receiving empathy express feelings of acceptance, caring, and value by others. When this is practiced there seems to be a strengthening of connectivity to people of the organizations. For an example, when a colleague models empathetic behavior, there could be a reward that recognizes the colleague for this behavior. This reinforces the behavior and also builds connectivity between the colleague and the organization.

Our Work Families

Unfortunately, sometimes colleagues may feel their daily work tasks are the only important thing valued by leadership. Leaders on the other hand, may feel that colleagues do not appreciate the fact that they have a job and the many efforts that leadership takes daily to give them the opportunity of work.

The bottom line is this: both the organization and the colleague need each other. It is essentially a work marriage. In the majority of occupations, this work marriage clocks many more waking hours with each other than in a traditional marital or family relationship. For example, an colleague who works a 40 hour work week spends eight hours on the job and a certain amount of time driving to her/his work that may add another two hours of travel time. This equates to ten hours dedicated to work life a day. The worker has to sleep, so this would equate to approximately seven hours a sleep. This results in seventy percent of an employee's time obligated to work and sleep during the Monday-Friday work week. Out of a twenty four hour day, this leaves thirty percent of time to devote to family or activities that are fulfilling to a colleague. Colleagues spend the majority of their waking hours with their co-workers at their workplace. Children's sports competitions and performances, parenting and household commitments, and any hobbies or extracurricular activities all have to squeeze into the tiny space left in a worker's life.

My husband and I while raising our two children had approximately 1.5-2 hours to talk during the five day work week as we prepared ourselves for bed and tried to unwind from our day. A similar scenario plays out daily in many American homes. Additional demands on the life of workers can come from a variety of things, such as extended commutes, longer shifts of work expected, overtime to cover co-worker absences, aging parent demands, and a million other things. The list is basically endless.

Life can be tough, demanding and draining. Is there any wonder why energy drinks are flying off the shelves? So the employee arrives at work and in many cases feels that their leadership and or management only desires to work them into the ground so the organization can make a large profit? Ouch, that stings. But there just may be some truth in this. Colleagues are the core of any organization and we as leaders and managers must have empathy for them as human beings and not treat them like a commodity, tools for accomplishing tasks, or a budget line item.

What Keeps Leadership from Empathy

I understand that a lack of empathy is often unintentional by leaders and managers. I truly understand the challenges and complexities related to the role of a healthcare leader. But I do believe there are problems associated with the deficit of empathy in healthcare today. There are hundreds of reasons and excuses that sound fairly legitimate for not taking the necessary steps or time to connect, value, and demonstrate empathy toward colleagues. But that does not make it the correct or admirable leadership trait. First, the leader must wholeheartedly believe the practice of empathy is important and possess this as a core value within their leadership philosophy. It must be part of the leadership agenda. It is clearly up to each leader and manager to be intentional and create time and space in their leadership agenda to achieve this. Empathy is not something that can be "delegated" to someone else. There will need to be support for this type of cultural environment in the senior and middle management staff, as well as support from governing boards.

Like so many people working in other positions, this leader may be working in a job that is not in their strength zone. If this is the case, the leader will stay conflicted and frustrated and others around them will feel the same. If a healthcare leader does not possess the competency and values of interpersonal relationships, then this can create major problems in a people industry like healthcare.

If you do not currently possess the interpersonal empathy skills you need, seek them. Anyone can develop and improve in this area. Whether you want to succeed in leadership or simply to thrive at work; developing yourself in this area will greatly increase your success.

Practicing Empathy

Empathizing with others requires self-reflection. Self-reflection allows us to become aware of how our actions affect others. The emphasis is not on our wants and needs but on the other person needs. In our highly self-centered world, we are often fully focused on our personal agendas and goals. There definitely appears to be a great need to study empathy in America and around the world. In fact, from listening to and reading news media stories on a regular basis it seems empathy could be one of the most important words for our world in this decade.

Empathy helps us not be self-centered, greedy and self-absorbed. It connects people's hearts. When we are empathetic, we seek to understand people more, resulting in more compassionate behavior. Empathy has also been said to sensitize the heart. The same is true with the workplace, if there is not intentional emphasis on the cultivation of an environment that has empathy as a core value it will not naturally exist. This is why empathy awareness for colleagues has to be a top priority of leadership for the organization.

A core organizational practice of fostering, modeling, and demonstrating an environment of empathy in the workplace will be worth the investment. Over many years in healthcare, I became increasingly aware of the need for practicing colleague empathy. In response, I developed a mastermind group session on the topic of empathy with some of my model colleague (who I refer to as my "Soaring Eagles"). By the end of the session, many colleagues were sharing how one or more fellow colleague had supported them in regard to a problem or issue they were having outside of their work. In one situation, the stress of going through a marital separation, the concern expressed by their colleague made all the difference in the way they were feeling. The empathy shared helped them make it through the day and accomplish their work. By the close of my mastermind session some of the colleagues were brought to tears simply by mentioning their empathy experiences. Working with people who care was monumental to them. Working with leaders that authentically cared about them made them feel valued, safe and appreciated.

Keep it Simple

Shared empathy creates a space between two people who they can identify with one another's feelings. It may be something as simple as pulling for the same team in sports, identifying with each other's enjoyment of a hobby or pastime, common child-raising or aging parent care experiences, an aspect of similar jobs, similar background or birthplaces. This creates a common connection that develops bonds in relationships.

Empathy can be shared by one person to another and from one person to many. A healthcare supervisor could show empathy to a group of healthcare colleagues who are working overtime due to the fact they have experienced this them self. The supervisor could demonstrate their empathy by furnishing a snack for the colleagues because they understand they are being delayed leaving work and getting an evening meal. The manager knows how this feels. The colleague sacrifices are self-reflected by the manager and motivate the manager to extend kindness and appreciation to the colleagues because they know how the colleagues are feeling. Demonstrating empathy is not difficult when you begin to truly walk in someone else's shoes.

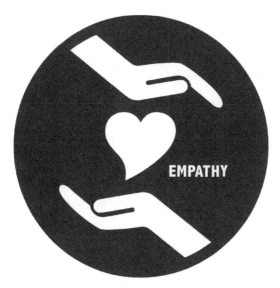

Figure 5

Our Empathy Symbol

The Corporate Transcendence™ Empathy Symbol[xxvi] is a visual representation of the way empathy is created between two people. In it, you see two hands reaching toward one another, creating between them an environment of value, caring, and love. Sometimes the two hands represent the hands of a caregiver and a patient. At others, they represent the hands of two colleagues. Empathy can only be created in your environment by reaching toward others, seeking to understand, and choosing to care about – and care for – the hearts of others. Because empathy is central to the healthcare experience, look for ways to recognize empathy among all colleagues and provide the visual reminder to practice empathy at all times.

Culture Transformation Action Steps:

Frontline Staff:
In the "gloved world" of modern healthcare, never underestimate the power of a kind word, smile, or touch. Eye contact, soft hand on the shoulder, and encouraging words can make a great difference. The greatest emotion that the majority of patients and their loved ones will experience in healthcare is fear. Remember patients are not interested in how busy you are or how much you know until they know how much you care.

Managerial Leadership:
Listening can be a greater act of empathy than talking. When your frontline colleagues arrive to work, remember that they bring an interactive life with them, such as relationships with spouses, children, family and friends. They come with their own unique set of personal challenges and problems. Managerial leadership can practice empathy by valuing their colleagues and demonstrating genuine interest in their lives. When a colleague has a problem and it is brought to you, it is usually a concern that could not be solved at the direct care front. This becomes management's role to listen and clarify with empathetic questioning. A key component of management's empathy model is to listen, care, encourage, and pitch in and help when needed.

Executive Leadership:
Leadership has the responsibility to recognize the importance of genuine empathy demonstrated toward their colleagues for optimal organizational efficiency. If empathy is a focus of leaders and the walk and talk align, it will be more of a focus by caregivers toward each other and the patients

they care for. About 80% of leadership actions should involve listening and seeking to understand. The remaining 20% goes to executing solutions or making changes. Your empathy model at this level involves having a higher awareness to stay tuned into the realities being faced at each level of the organizations and being proactive in meeting the human's needs of patients and colleagues.

CHAPTER 7

Ownership: The Best of Self

• • •

"We can change the world and make it a better place. It is in your hands to make a difference."

Nelson Mandela

Defining Ownership

Ownership is a powerful blend of personal responsibility and self-efficacy; not only are we responsible for ourselves and the environment we help facilitate, but every individual is fully capable of making a positive difference in their life and others. Regardless of your situation or job position, there is always something in your work that you can do to reinforce or influence what is happening around you, Ownership does not mean owning only what is written in your job description. Ownership means never hiding behind the statement of "that isn't my job," or "I shouldn't have to." Expressing ownership means investing the best of you to get the best out of your organization. Your attitudes and mindset have an incredible impact on the organization and the people around you. Colleagues should think of themselves as the chiefs of their area and beyond. Colleagues need to understand that their day-to-day decisions have a direct effect on the business success in finance, culture, quality and governance.

This mindset will work its way down to the patient. Colleagues will find themselves thinking "if this was my mother, how would I want her to be treated?" as well as "if this was my budget, how would I use this money?" Colleagues treasure, look after and tend to those things of which they feel ownership. Owning something is a privilege. Colleagues honor that privilege by investing in the organization they work for every day by the way they own their work.

THE POWER OF ONE

There is not a single great thing accomplished on earth that has only one person responsible for it. It takes the combination of many people to achieve something amazing and notable. But one person can have an idea or hold a belief within him to do more, be more, give more and make a difference in the world. The power of one person should never be underestimated. The power that one person possesses can result in positive or negative outcomes in this world. This fact has been seen repeatedly through history. World changers like Nelson Mandela, Abraham Lincoln, Margaret Thatcher, and Mother Teresa all had one thing in common: ownership that led to significance in the world.

Other massively influential individuals have exerted the "power of one" include Heinrich Himmler, Jeffrey Dahmer, Saddam Hussein, and Adolf Hitler. People with bad intentions, as well as people with great intentions, have made a negative or positive difference in the world. There is no doubt the world needs more people exhibiting ownership with the desire to be a positive influence. We need people courageous and bold enough to declare a mission and cast their vision within their world to make a significant difference where they live and beyond.

THE POWER SOURCE

Power that fuels greatness comes from within the minds, heart, and souls of people. People who have made a difference have been people who consciously and intentionally made the decision to step forward and do something that they feel is needed or called to do. Many times there is a consistent tug within them, a dream to do more and become more. They have a passion burning within them that cannot be quenched. It comes from the depths of their very being. It gives them strength and power.

The internal desire to make a difference outweighs any necessary requirements for additional work, energy, time, sacrifice and resources that may have to be expended. Their motivation and power to move forward as an individual is driven by the need to make a significant difference in the world in which they live. There is an intentional mindset not to accept something the way it is but to improve or change it. A healthcare colleague's feeling of being able to actually fulfill a need or void in patient's lives is self-edifying. When repeated, most the time it creates higher energy that builds momentum for the mission.

The willingness to step up to a worthy mission will also draw other people to follow the cause. Take for example the Susan G. Komen Foundation. This organization was formed from the passion of Susan's sister to prevent and eradicate breast cancer after watching her sister lose her battle to this tragic disease. Susan G. Komen Foundation has raised millions of dollars and saved thousands of lives through their mammography screening programs for early detection of breast cancer. This is a high profile example of the power of one from the personal experience of pain to make a difference in the world.

Each day in healthcare, there are many opportunities and specific moments in time for us to make a positive difference for others. It could be a word or act of encouragement. It could be meeting a need in the community or for family members. It may be doing something to improve the work environment or operations. A healthcare colleague once shared with me how she routinely pays the expense of the meal of the person behind her in the fast food line. She does this to encourage others and hope that she is an example that inspires others to help one another. Something simple like that is a statement both of valuing people, and taking consistent action to build others up. Leo Buscagla states "Too often we underestimate the power of a touch, a smile, a kind word, a listening ear, an honest compliment, or the smallest act of caring, all of which have the potential to turn a life around."

The power of one in the healthcare environment is having the mindset not to succumb to status quo or mediocrity, seeking instead to improve things for their organization, colleagues, and patients they care for. We tap into the power of one when we consciously engage in the lives of our patients and colleagues, and choose to improve our environment to make it positive, regardless of adverse circumstances or potential barriers.

The power of one is strong enough to start a revolution toward positive change in the workplace or world and should never be underestimated. Each person has the power of one through their ability, talents, strengths, and beliefs.

INFLUENCE IS POWER – POSITIVE OR NEGATIVE

The power to influence is in everyone. This power can manifest or be suppressed. The power of one can be positive or negative and can result in a positive or negative influence or impact on other people and situations. The influencing power of positivity can be contagious, just like the power of negativity. If we desire to be a positive influencer, we will seek ways to learn, grow and model our life in this way. We will participate in activities that positively impact our lives and others.

People who chose to be a negative influence will seek ways to be destructive and cause conflict and chaos. People have power and power has influence. A person who is on a team to complete a project and is dominating and controlling is wielding their power to influence the team in a desirable way that may not be best for the team. This type of behavior is seen as negative because a team is supposed to hear all members' viewpoints and share in decision making. The behavior of this one person is seen as negative to the team and creates dysfunction within the team.

With the many clocked hours colleagues spend at work, the influence felt by our colleagues is very important. The many personal decisions made each minute directly impact their environment ranging from poor to good to great. Each individual possess ownership of their influence. Colleagues must hold themselves accountable for the ways they chose to affect their environment. Each person has inherent power to lead others by their influence. Parents do this every day. They can lead their children in the way they should behave through teaching and modeling behaviors. A colleague can lead them self by opening up their life to positive influences. The more positive influencing people that surround a person, the more positive and encouraged they become. Living and leading life in an intentional and positive manner will yield positive thinking and thoughts that lead to behaviors. What a person chooses to put into their mind is what comes out in their words and actions.

POWER OF ONE IS NOT A THREAT

How much influence people desire is determined by the individual? I have observed many healthcare colleagues who feel that they have limited power, and underestimate their power to influence others. There are a number of reasons a person may feel this way. Maybe it is because of their life experiences, their home environment, early upbringing, or simply the cultural norm where they work. In working with many colleagues through the years, many people feel inadequate to voice an opinion at work even when they feel it will make their work or organization better.

Those who feel they lack influence are often taken off guard when their leaders, managers, and supervisors ask for their opinions. They normally do not feel their thoughts are valued so they do not voice them. There is a lack of understanding in the power of one and their influence, when this is not the expectation of the culture in which they work. Transforming the culture to one of valuing their voice and influence can truly transform an organization.

POWER OF ONE – THE PATIENT

In March 2002, The Joint Commission – together with the Centers for Medicare and Medicaid Services – launched a national campaign to urge patients to take a role in preventing healthcare errors by becoming active, involved, and informed participants on their healthcare team. Speak Up™ encourages patients to:

* Speak up if you have questions or concerns. If you still do not understand, ask again. It is your body and you have a right to know.
* Pay attention to the care you get. Always make sure you're getting the right treatments and medicines by the right healthcare professionals. Never assume.
* Educate yourself about your illness. Learn about the medical tests you get, and your treatment plan.
* Ask a trusted family member or friend to be your advocate (advisor or supporter).
* Know what medicines you take and why you take them. Medicine errors are the most common healthcare mistakes.
* Use a hospital, clinic, surgery center, or other type of healthcare organization that has been carefully checked out. For example, The Joint Commission visits hospitals to see if they are meeting The Joint Commission's quality standards.
* Participate in all decisions about your treatment. You are the center of the healthcare team.

Speak Up – Colleagues

A similar campaign can be used in a healthy organizational culture for colleagues. Healthcare colleagues should be encouraged to speak up and participate in decision making, process improvement, and problem solving. People who do the work each day feel valued for their contributions and are encouraged to speak up and share thoughts and ideas on how to improve their work processes and the organization. Some leaders may view the encouragement of workers to use their thoughts and opinions and voice power and influence as a threat, even as acts of insubordination. If this is the case, it presents a leadership problem that needs to be addressed. It takes all healthcare colleagues working together to deliver the best care to patients possible.

POWER OF ONE – BARRIERS

Traditionally, healthcare has been a more formal culture that fosters a ranking and a superiority mentality. Culture driven only from the top down does not promote individuality or fully recognize the power of colleagues' influence on the organization. Leaders and colleagues in this environment will admit that little is known about colleagues beyond what their clinical certification or license represents, or the department they work in or who they report to. This mindset is dangerous and deadly to the organization as well as the patients served. It can create a closed communication system that yields expectations of underperformers. Healthcare leaders and colleagues must recognize that two heads are always better than one, and three heads are always better than two. Healthcare environments function well when there is a partnership among all caregivers who model a sense of valuing and respect for each other. In such an environment colleagues may support one another, sharing their best with each other, so that the patient and organization can deliver superior care.

Traditionally, influencers have been thought to be the people in the organization with the most authority, the individuals with the special titles, job authority, and the power. Influence coming from other colleagues in the organization was not considered to be significant unless it met the approval of those with the title, authority, and power. Many colleagues have the perspective that it is only the title that will allow them to have true influence on others. The titled persons may be the force that primarily drives influence in the organization, but in a culture of excellence, influence is provided by all colleague stakeholders. Everyone has ownership, a voice, with the right to be heard and valued for their input in order to make the organization the best it can become.

In environments where only the leadership possesses ownership, it is dangerous. Soloing problem solving by isolating departments crushes innovation, creativity, and learning. If there are five people in the room having a discussion, then there are five opinions and perspectives to consider. Viewing a topic from a variety of perspectives enriches the discussion and can create new ideas which expand and can enlighten the thinking of the people in the room. Fostering the power of individual thinking shared among groups, allows ideas to manifest thoughts and "outside of the box" thinking can easily occur. Creative, imaginative and critical independent thinking is a great mental exercise for an individual who desires to build influence inside or out of a team setting.

SUPPORTING THE DEVELOPMENT OF ONE'S POWER

It cannot be assumed that colleagues always have the competencies necessary to perform their responsibilities optimally. In healthcare, like most industries, it takes the ongoing commitment of leadership for colleague education to help them remain equipped with what they must have to be successful. If they choose to continue their professional education outside the organization by earning an additional degree or certification, that should be celebrated by an organization that believes that each colleague personally contributes to a culture of excellence.

When colleagues develop themselves personally, they improve their ability to use their influence for good within an organization. This can be something as simple as improving interpersonal communication skills, or as complex as getting an advanced degree. Ownership means that colleagues can choose at any time to find some way to develop themselves, and thereby expand their influence. Ownership also means that colleagues choose to use all of their education and experiences as they go about their work and they feel accountable to the quality of work they produce. Colleagues make a conscious decision to choose to "show up, filled up" daily to work. That means colleagues need to bring all of their abilities to work, taking responsibility for their actions and their environment, and positively grows their influence in order to give their best to the organization.

THE SIGNIFICANCE OF YOU

The significance of YOU, as the healthcare worker includes everyone from the housekeeper, phlebotomist, doctor, nurse, chief executive officer, physical therapist, patient transport, nutritionist, surgical nurse, imaging technologist, and the countless other roles within the health-care world. All healthcare colleagues hold vastly important roles to en-sure the success of our industry. Think of each colleague as number one in importance to healthcare success. Just imagine what it would be like not to have environmental services cleaning and taking care of the health environment. Imagine all the dangerous microorganisms lurking around and growing into a large reservoir of life-threatening viruses and bacteria. We all know a microorganism can live in the smallest drop of body fluid and gain entrance into the body through the tiniest paper cut, multiplying quickly and moving through the bloodstream. Just think of the Ebola virus. In Ebola infections, the patient's blood is infected with a deadly microorganism that will turn the blood toxic and in the major-ity of cases causes' death. This creates blood that kills, instead of blood that heals.

The same thing can be said for the workplace culture of healthcare or-ganizations. Our organization can become a culture that heals or a culture that kills. Just as our blood gives each of one of us life, a colleague con-tributes to the life and health of their organization. The culture produced is capable of healing or killing. People make up the culture. A healthy culture begins with relationships and must be developed, protected, nur-tured, and cared for daily. Just as a deadly virus can infect the body, a sick or toxic culture can infect the organization and become deadly to the or-ganization and its mission.

A Person's Influential Power as a Team Member

Teamwork is an imperative base on which our new model of America healthcare will operate. A patient-centric healthcare model requires a host of caregivers to wrap around services that meet the needs of the patient in a holistic manner. All factors of a person's being come into account. For example the patient's social, physical, mental, dental, and financial needs all must be examined to deliver the best health possible. Success for the patient's clinical outcome can only be achieved through a team caregiver model where there is accountability for the influence that each team and team delivers successful care to the patient.

The power of a team is absolutely greater than the power of one, but a team is at its strongest when the individuals on the team bring their best values, competencies, and strengths to the table. There is a saying that "one bad apple will spoil the whole bushel," and over time this is true. Also unfortunately, that will be the case if an individual brings negative values, poor competencies, and weak efforts to the team. If you have been on a team and witnessed some of these issues, you know exactly how this can derail the team. We would be wise to never take the power of one lightly. Each colleague impacts the outcomes a team can achieve for itself and for the organization as a whole. On a broad scale, leadership values the power of one by carefully choosing every team member.

The Dream Team

Taking ownership does not mean becoming the Lone Ranger. Moving personal perspectives from "me" thing to a "team" thing should be a part of daily role modeling and influencing from leadership and management. A team member who exhibits high functionality contributes to the creation of the "Dream Team." "Dream Team" members value each other and appreciate their complementary strengths and propel their team and organization to success.

Colleagues need to feel personal satisfaction in their work. Building strong teams begins with valuing their own significant contribution as well as the contributions of each team member. The collective strengths of a team, regardless of their role, can make a creditable difference in the team and its quality. A hospital facility worker works with his or her team in keeping the facility operating at its best. Facility services, environmental services, and the operative services staff work as a team to ensure the surgical suites are sterile and operating optimally at all times. Operative suites must have perfect heating, ventilation and air conditioning. This is as much a part of saving lives as the surgical procedure. A poorly functioning environmental surgical climate could create a detrimental atmosphere for a patient.

Appreciating the work of an individual or team can be demonstrated in a number of ways, by colleagues, managers, and leaders. One powerful way to do this is to recognize and commend teams and colleagues when something outstanding is accomplished, or excellent work is done. Doing this in the eyes of peers adds significance impact to the recognition, and is an important part of valuing. While it is important to emphasize appropriate attention and care for the patient, leaders must understand it is just as important to demonstrate care amongst colleagues.

TEAMS DELIVER

Team performance impacts the viability of the mission, vision, values, behavioral creed, and the overall organization's performance. Success is only sustainable when teams effectively work together. Participation and communication is essential to keeping the strategic focus of the team in check. Leaders are particularly influential.

As leaders, we must continually remind ourselves and our colleagues how valuable each of us are to the success of the organization. Through personal education and the development of colleagues and teams, they become more sensitive to the needs of the organization and their focus becomes more of how they will benefit the organization versus a what-is-in-it-for-me attitude.

ATTITUDES

Behaviors and attitudes go hand in hand because they are driven by thoughts and beliefs. Attitudes are played out in actions that result in what others perceive as an individual's character. Attitudes may align or contrast with the organizational culture. Attitudes determined to be best for the organization by leadership must be communicated clearly to provide guidance in behaviors to all colleagues. Attitudes matter and cannot be taken for granted. Attitudes embraced in healthcare have to be intentional.

As individuals, we have to set a governor on our attitude and constantly be reminded of the attitude that we need to embrace, in order to be successful in our life and work. To have a good attitude in life, a person must elect to have a positive mindset. A positive mindset leads to a positive attitude. If we want to develop a positive organizational culture, there also must be a mindset that all colleagues' behaviors make a difference.

LEADERSHIP MINDSET

I would like you to repeat something. Say it out loud. Do not worry about what others may think. Just declare "I am a leader! "How did this declaration make you feel? All colleagues should think of themselves as the Chief Executive Officer of themselves and their work. You are the Chief of you! This mindset of personal authority is powerful in helping an individual feel they have influence and control over their work experience. What do you think it would be like if the leaders and all colleagues in your organization treated each person like they were the CEO of their particular job?

Let's look at David, who is part of the Environment Services Department, who is responsible for cleaning the floors. The floor tech usually reports to a manager who creates a schedule and provides the necessary resources for the floor tech to do their job effectively. It is the floor tech; however, who leads the actual process of cleaning the floors and has influence on the minor details related to how the job is performed. This floor tech does not have any employees who report to him, but the truth is that David is leading himself, and it influencing all of his own decisions for the day. David is the CEO of his job. If we can convince each colleague that leadership is not about title, experience, or degree, but about influencing your mindset, then we will have empowered colleagues. Empowered colleagues feel pride in their work; take initiative, and are accountable for their tasks. They use their self-leadership for the betterment of the organization: consider the quote from Martin Luther King, Jr. "If a man is called to be a street sweeper, he should sweep streets even as Michelangelo painted, or Beethoven composed music, or Shakespeare wrote poetry. He should sweep streets so well that all the host of heaven and earth will pause to say, "Here lived a great street sweeper who did his job well."

This concept may be difficult to grasp for some people because it involves placing power in the hands of colleagues that do not officially have a leadership "title." From a young age, we have been programmed to think that a leader is someone with an important title. Even, in our home lives, individual influence and authority is demonstrated greatly in roles as a mother, father, caregiver, and provider. As a leader, would you rather have 50 staff members taking personal responsibility for their position as if they were the CEO of their work, or would you rather have all of the responsibility fall on a few individuals' shoulders?

Everyone is a leader. When I state this to frontline colleagues, it usually takes a period of time to process. When you lead yourself, you influence others. Leaders should encourage all colleagues to think of themselves as CEO of their work – to "be the CEO of YOU." This mindset of having authority is powerful in helping colleagues feel that they can influence their work experience. All people known as influencers who use their positions for the betterment of an organization should be known as great leaders.

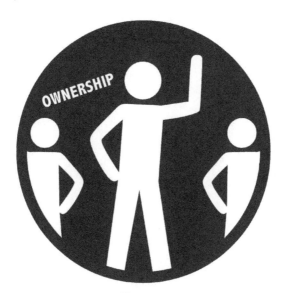

Figure 6

Our Ownership Symbol

The Corporate Transcendence™ Ownership Symbol[xxviii] illustrates the importance of standing up, using your voice, and actively taking action in creating the best work environment possible. This symbol demonstrates a single person standing, when others are not. This is to show that there are many things individuals can do, without waiting on others to join in. Regardless of position or title, a person is never truly powerless. This symbol represents the action of ownership, implying an empowered mindset and sense of responsibility to do what we can in any given situation to make it the best it can possibly be.

Culture Transformation Action Steps:

Frontline Staff:

Taking ownership of the work environment by the front line is the most powerful transformation factor in your organization. Your behavior in modeling ownership of work responsibility has a direct impact on your patient care, and colleague interaction. Expressing ownership at the front line can have as much or ultimately more overall influence on the organization as compared to the CEO! You are on stage for every behavior you display, your attitude, and conversation. What you do will color the environment around you. You as one brings influence to people's lives. Own your talents and develop your leadership abilities regardless of your title, position or job. You are the gatekeeper to your destiny.

Managerial Leadership:

Foster and encourage the strengths of your frontline staff so they are engaged and take ownership of their work in an effective way that can make a greater positive difference. Maintain colleagues' involvement so that they see themselves as part of the solution and not the problem. Recognize the value of team activities. Show that their attitudes, behaviors, and excellence matter by specifically recognizing and thanking them for using their gifts. The peer influence on the culture of ownership is massive. Keep your eye out for the skills and gifts of your frontline staff so that you can utilize and leverage them.

Executive Leadership:

Ownership at the executive level means working for the organization first and not self. The executive leader has to see the big picture without forgetting that details matter – it is not just the big stuff that is big stuff. Ownership is not about owning the TITLE. It is about owning the VISION. Be a full expression of what the organization values, its mission and vision. There is no room for ego at this level; be approachable.

CHAPTER 8

Personal Strengths: Cultivating High Performance

• • •

*"You cannot have faith in people unless you take
action to inspire and develop them."*

SUMANTRA GHOSHAL

DEFINING PERSONAL STRENGTHS

Personal strengths are the inborn attributes that make each person a master-piece. Each individual must recognize they possess unique strengths and the importance of their own personal strengths to their life. The best investment one could make in themselves, family, friends, employer, and colleagues is to develop their natural strengths. Healthcare organizations that recognize and embrace every colleague's strengths help colleagues to understand themselves. Utilizing these strengths to the benefit of the organization helps it to achieve its mission and vision. The cumulative power of maximizing strengths will make an incredible difference in all areas of the organization.

THE LATE EMPLOYEE

Susan was late for work...every single day. Her manager "spoke" with her several times, and eventually gave her a written warning for her tardiness.

The week after the written warning, she was late on three separate occasions. Her manager "had enough" and was ready to terminate Susan, a new marketing assistant in the hospital's public relations department.

Thankfully, Susan's manager (Rob) had a conversation with a talent manager (Sarah) that went something like this:

Rob: "I'm done with Susan. She's been late for work three times this week, and I just wrote her up. Doesn't she get it?"

Sarah: "Yes, that's frustrating. I can see it's upsetting you. What would you like to do?"

Rob: "I'm thinking we should move forward right away with some type of progressive discipline. She needs to know she should follow policy when I ask her to change her behavior."

Sarah: "So you don't think Susan takes you seriously?"

Rob: "Well, no....she does....on most things, but obviously not as it relates to her chronic tardiness."

Sarah: "I want to support you Rob, and I can tell that it seems like Susan is not respecting your wishes, but before we move forward I just have a couple of questions, is that ok?"

Rob: "Sure, I welcome any thoughts you have."

Sarah: "Well first of all, do you know why Susan is late? Have you asked her?"

Rob: "Ummm...well...no. I guess I haven't asked her that directly."

Sarah: "Is that something you could do this week to try and learn more about Susan, to show you care about her situation, and to try and possibly problem solve with her?"

Rob: "Sure. I don't see what difference it will make but I can try."

Sarah: "Ok, great. Let me know how it goes, and I'll be happy to support you or give feedback. My other question was related to Susan's job performance. How is it? What are her strengths?"

Rob: "Well, she's only been here four weeks, but the new social media plan she put together is outstanding. The quality of her work is really top notch, she gets along really well with everyone, but it's like she just doesn't..."

Sarah: "Ok....so her work is excellent. You are happy with her actual work performance right now."

Rob: "Actually, yes, very much so. I guess I've been so focused on her being late that I've been so frustrated to really even think much about her work quality."

Sarah: "I get it. Because she doesn't arrive on time like you requested, you feel a lack of respect and feel less respect toward her in return. But essentially you have a good colleague on your hands that seems to be a good fit for the job in many other ways. If she has excellent marketing skills, and gets along well with her coworkers, how important is it that she arrives to work at a certain time?"

Rob: "Well, it's just the principle of it. She's being disrespectful."

Sarah: "Ok, well if you could put that aside for a second, and try not to take her tardiness as a personal attack, is it really that important for her to arrive at 8:00am on the dot?"

Rob: "Well, I guess not. I mean she needs to get a certain amount of work done every day. But I guess technically it doesn't really matter when she arrives to work if I think about it."

Sarah: "I totally agree. If we have a skilled employee with a good attitude on our hands, I just think we should try to find a way to keep her. Can you try to meet with her this week to understand the reasons why she is late, and come up with some type of plan that is mutually agreeable regarding her start time? Think outside the box? I bet it wouldn't hurt if she knew how you felt about her recent marketing campaign as well."

Rob: "Yeah, that sounds great. I can do that. I never really thought of myself as a strict manager, but I guess this timeliness thing is more important to me personally than it being a requirement of her job."

Sarah: "Awesome Rob. Thanks so much for exploring this with me. I'm just offering a different perspective. I know both of our goals are to retain talented colleagues and to work with their strengths. Let me know how it goes."

After his conversation with Talent Management, Rob scheduled a meeting with Susan. He empathized with her by asking why she was late every day. To Rob's surprise he learned that she had a special needs daughter who was one year old. This made it very difficult for Susan to get her ready by a set schedule each morning, drop her off at daycare, and get to work on time. Rob and Susan worked together to come up with a new plan that allowed Susan to arrive to work at 9:00am. Surprisingly, Susan made it to work on time for her new schedule every single day. Rob no longer felt disrespected because Susan always arrived on time. Susan seemed much happier because she didn't feel as stressed arriving to work, and didn't have to put as much pressure on her special needs child each morning. Something as simple as creating a later arrival time allowed her to utilize her strengths and flourish in the workplace. Susan's strengths in marketing shined.

Susan is now a tremendous asset to the marketing department, and a great asset to the hospital as a whole. That may not have been the case if a savvy talent management leader had not encouraged Rob to focus on Susan's strengths and value to the organization.

OUR GREATEST ASSETS

The truth is, colleagues like Susan are our greatest assets. Colleagues in every role and every position – from the highest responsibility to the lowest paid colleague – make the healthcare system function. All colleagues – no exceptions. On the other hand, colleagues can break an organization.

Colleagues can provide a great customer experience, or a terrible one. They can create best practices for quality care delivered to patients or provide poor quality of care. Colleagues can create a culture that heals, or a culture that can harm.

Colleagues ultimately hold the future success of healthcare in their hands. Leaders are dependent on what colleague strengths are, just as colleagues are dependent on what strengths their leaders possess. Colleagues will influence the culture, quality, and financial success of healthcare in every organization. Wise healthcare leaders embrace this fact. Leaders who can influence their colleagues by valuing and investing in their strengths will develop and propel the organization to its greatest potential.

The disappointing fact is that many people or colleagues do not truly understand their strengths. They settle for what they have experienced in life as their strengths from their past.

If a colleague was told in middle school that they are average in intelligence, their bar may get set there, and that is where they settle. People many times look externally for a new job, different colleagues or supervisor, a spouse or maybe having a child to make their life feel more valuable and meaningful. Sustaining fulfillment in life is found by focusing internally and by truly discovering and maximizing personal strengths and coming to understanding their unique purpose and passion in life. In our society, we often allow other people and life circumstances to define what a person may believe are their talents or strengths. This can result in self-limiting beliefs that are embraced by a person. Unfortunately it seems the world mirrors these beliefs. Challenging colleagues to revisit their beliefs about their strengths requires personal self-reflection. Thoughts about them and believing they possess certain strength, are two entirely different things. Thinking is a process and believing is action created by a transition in the mind. People need to be encouraged to explore and act on what they suspect or know their strengths to be.

WHY WE DENY OUR STRENGTHS

OUTWARD-FOCUS BIAS

Many times, when people are told they have strengths, their first reaction is to deny it. They may desire to believe, but their self-limiting beliefs kept them back from exploring these possible strengths. Most people are not encouraged to discover their strengths on an ongoing basis into adult years. People instead are trained to focus outward, this will constrict their strengths. A person may believe that their strengths as a person must come from an external, rather than internal source. An example would be to meet Prince Charming, have children and live the Cinderella dream. There is nothing wrong with these thoughts about meeting a great spouse or enjoying having children, but where in this story line do individuals begin to explore and value their own talents and strengths? Personal strengths should be enhanced by relationships, but not camouflaged by them. People need to discover and define their life by their natural strengths. Everyone possesses much strength to share in the world.

"INTELLIGENCE" LABELS

Maybe a person grew up believing that they would drop out of school and make minimum wage because this is the environment and behavior modeled in his or her life. Self-limiting beliefs about who we are and who we can become are just that: limiting.

In a historical 2008 research survey by New York sociologist, Patrick Sharkey and co-author Felix Elwert, surveyed thousands of American families and found that first generation of children that grew up in poor neighborhoods ran higher risk for ending up in poor neighborhoods as adults. When first generation became parents, this tendency for their children for living in poor neighborhoods continued. The study also showed that these families got less education, worse jobs, if any, and bear more physical, social and psychological problems.[xxix] There definitely seems to be a direct link between what is believed and a person's life.

Entertaining self-limiting thoughts are restrictive to the development and manifestation of an individual's inherent strengths. Limited thinking and beliefs leads to settling for less than our best. During my school years, we measured strengths by a grade received in a particular class. The belief was that you must be good at a subject if you received a good mark. The grade mark became a mental confirmation.

For example, if a student is told they have average intelligence in the eighth grade and that technical school versus college prep classes in high school is best for them, then very likely the student will easily buy into this belief. The belief can be even more destructive if it comes from a person of authority. Young children on the other hand believe in the extraordinary for their life. Children say they want to grow up to do and become amazing people like the President of the United States or a great lawyer, scientist, teacher, or doctor. They have not bought into the self-limiting beliefs at this development period of their life.

THE TRUTH ABOUT STRENGTHS

Strengths are part of who we are. They exist in our own DNA, given to us by our creator. Strengths are not rationed in anyway based on individual characteristics such as race, gender, socioeconomic status, who our parents were, or what we may have experienced in life. Individual DNA is unique to every human, just as his or her strengths are. Strengths should be discovered and celebrated in organizations by leaders and colleagues. It is like setting people free to be their best and do their best. The process of identifying and unleashing colleague strengths is powerful and will elevate the organization to new heights. Living at the core of every organization are the strengths. Developing the strengths of this core will create excellence and transcendence for the organization.

CHICKENS & EAGLES

I once heard a great story about engaging the DNA strengths of colleagues from a teacher. The following is my version of the story:

Chickens & Eagles

Once there was an eagle that was living on a farm and grew up among chickens in a chicken coop. Day after day he walked, talked, ate, and squawked like the chickens. The eagle saw himself as a mirror image of the chickens he lived with. One day as he was looking up at the sky, he saw a very large bird with wide-spread wings, soaring high above the chicken coop. The eagle eagerly asked the chickens what kind of bird was in the sky. The chickens told him that was an eagle. The eagle said to the chickens, "I want to be an eagle!" The chickens squawked and squawked, belly laughing, and cried out to the eagle, "You are not an eagle silly, you are a chicken! You cannot fly like that eagle. You have to stay down here with us as a chicken." As days went by, month after month, the eagle would cast eyes at the eagle soaring across the sky and repeat to himself, "I am an eagle, I am an eagle."

The eagle's circumstances said to him that he was a chicken, but deep down in his being he felt he was an eagle. As the eagle grew to be older he decided that he was going to try to fly like the eagle. Being a chicken had been ingrained into him, but he did not want to settle for average, he wanted to be more. So one day with all the courage he could muster inside himself, the eagle walked to the edge of the chicken coop and carefully planned his next upward moves across the chicken yard. The eagle raised and stretched his wings as high as he could and began to run as fast as he could, flapping his wings as hard as he possibly could. He began to lift off the ground and in a brief moment he began to feel that he was an eagle and he could truly fly. Then as quickly as the feeling came, it left. He flew directly into the side of the chicken coup and crashed to the ground, rolling to an exhausting halt. He lay there motionless casting his eyes to the big blue sky.

The chickens observing the entire disastrous flight began to laugh uncontrollably with so much noise that it made all the animals in the barnyard join in. All the chickens began to shout at the same time, telling the eagle how stupid he was to think he could fly. The eagle slowly stood up under the roar of the crowded chicken yard and walked slowly with his head hung low to the corner of the yard and buried his head into one of his wings. Broken-hearted and feeling defeated, the eagle felt like a total failure and started blaming himself for his failed flight, repeating to himself over and over, "How could I ever think that I could be an eagle? I am not an eagle, I am a chicken!"

For many days and weeks following the failed flight, the eagle began to look forward to catching the image of the beautiful, graceful eagle soaring with its outstretched wings high above the trees tops. He would strain his neck upward with his eyes focused for as long as the eagle was in his sight, studying each detail of the eagle's movements. He evaluated every delicate angle and lift of the eagle's wings as he soared high above the clouds and dipped gracefully across the canvas of the blue sky. Day after day he admired and studied the eagle. He began to anticipate the bodily movement of the eagle and he felt as if he was along the eagle's side flying with total freedom without feeling the fence caging him. Then upon arising to a new day, he walked into the chicken yard looking at the beautiful blue sky, and then back to the chickens that were picking the ground around the yard.

The eagle looked again to the sky and began to repeat to himself: "I am not a chicken, I am an eagle! I am not a chicken, I am an EAGLE! I am not a chicken, I am an eagle! I was created to be an eagle. An eagle is what I was created to be!" Then, with wings outstretched, he began to move just as he had seen the soaring eagle so many times before. Suddenly his body began to rise from the ground as graceful as if it had done so thousands of times before. He rose higher and higher and was flying above the chicken yard when the chickens below stopped pecking and looked up in disbelief. He rose higher and higher among the clouds of the vast sky and became the eagle he was born to be.

YOUR HIDDEN EAGLES

Many employees will come to you with the mindset of being less than their best. They will succumb to negative social influence and mirror the actions of their peers. They will not recognize their individual strengths, talents, or uniquely-designed gifts. Organizations with a culture of valuing employees will help them to discover their strengths that will transform many colleagues into eagles, and help connect each individual to the personal and unique DNA of his or her greatness.

We have established that colleagues are an organization's most valuable asset. Each of these valuable assets possesses strengths unique to them. Utilizing and valuing these strengths will give an organization an advantage on others. Ignoring these strengths will be a barrier to organizational success and bring forth a host of unnecessary problems. Problems such as high turnover, low morale, and inconsistent job performance are just a few. Another great way to look at personal strengths is like diamonds hidden in a yard, waiting to be discovered. But because the diamonds are unknown, one may never guess to dig or look for them. Our colleague's strengths are like diamonds scattered in a yard, waiting to be discovered. Leaders need to remember that discovering and sustaining the sparkle requires intentional cultural strategic development and planning.

A CULTURE OF VALUING

We have all heard the rule airlines teach: "Secure your own oxygen mask before assisting others." In healthcare, this means helping our colleague first, before turning our efforts toward our patients. First, place the oxygen mask on our colleagues, so they can deliver their best in providing care to patients. Doing this requires investing time, money, resources, and energy into each colleague, then the investment will yield later more time, money, resources and energy for the organization. Many healthcare leaders may feel that we cannot afford to do this. My response: healthcare leaders cannot afford NOT to do this to meet the demands of today's healthcare industry.

Most of the educations for colleagues in healthcare are related to training that is specific to a new policy or procedure, sponsored and encouraged by a regulatory agency that drives delivery of care. These types of training are imperative, but this training alone does not transform a culture. These trainings are very structured and reveal rules, guidelines, or procedures that need to be followed and maintained. Unfortunately, I have seen these types of repeated training drain colleagues and place great pressure, anxiety and a fear of failing. Fear and insecurity may lurk in their minds because they cannot remember every important detail to the thousands of policies and regulations. Leaders must create a healthy culture of valuing colleagues to keep this energy in balance. If not, colleagues feel overburdened and taken advantage of. Leaders suffer with the same fears that colleagues struggle with, though perhaps in slightly different ways. Creating a culture of valuing eliminates the fear of failing and replaces it with an attitude of understanding and "failing forward." A culture of valuing does not mean perfection, but rather a desire to exceed expectations and continue positive momentum.

A culture of valuing means creating learning opportunities from best practices and preventable errors. A healthy culture is a proactive culture, continuously scanning the horizon looking for opportunities to improve and excel. This cannot be accomplished by a few people, all colleagues must participate. A valuing culture cultivates all colleagues to higher levels of engagement.

The day of leaders being "everything to everybody" is over. Leaders, you can sit down and take a breath. Your job is to lead, foster, and orchestrate the organization into excellence by utilizing your greatest strengths to the best of your ability. As a leader, recruit diamonds and continue to discover and value their strengths. Leaders must allow their diamonds to sparkle and watch them lead the organization up to the summit of success. As a healthcare leader, this is one of the most rewarding experiences to observe.

A healthy culture is rich in colleagues utilizing their strengths to move the organization higher than colleagues or leaders ever thought possible. When colleagues are in their strength zones, they naturally raise the performance bar and expect to grow toward the next rung of the personal and professional ladder. They become engaged and empowered colleagues, who will settle for nothing less. They live in the belief that their contributions build excellence; they hold the expectation that their organization's next BEST, will continually repeat itself.

THE IMPACT OF SURVEYS ON CULTURE

Historically, healthcare organizations are constantly and tirelessly preparing for inspections and surveys like The Joint Commission or maybe a Health Resource and Services Administration (HRSA) survey, or one of the many other local, state, and federal agencies that may come unannounced or scheduled to assess some aspect of the healthcare organization or facility. These surveys bring with them an incredible amount of work for ongoing regulatory compliance, accountability, and constant readiness.

There is education and training with staff anywhere from years to months to prepare to meet these demands. In many cases, due to changing guidelines, standards, and regulations on sometimes a monthly or an annual basis, leadership and management scramble to educate and train on new health polices and compliance standards. Constant bombardment of "we must do this or we will fail our inspection or survey" can be heard among colleagues as common remarks. This constant educational environment creates in many ways a fearful, "survival of the fittest" culture for colleagues. Fear of failing can lead to leaders or colleagues considering dishonesty as a strategy to avoid trouble or protect a sense of job security. One unfortunate example of this cultural thinking was witnessed on a national scale in 2014 when the Veterans Administration Hospital system shared that the wait times for Veterans to get a doctor's appointment was falsified to the government. According to the September 9, 2014, CBS Associated Press news article titled "VA Managers Lied About Problems, Inspector Says." Investigators said the efforts to cover up or hide the delays were systemic across the nearly 1,000 hospitals and clinics run by the VA.

When colleagues have the fear of failure, and feel challenged to perform adequately, this echoes in the halls and drains the energy from the environment. It creates a sick work environment. The valuing of strengths that are brought to the table by all respective colleagues will build a culture that brings the best out of the organization. This helps an organization pierce the veil of fear on surveys, instead performing with an excellence that flows from within each colleague. A healthy culture will find ways to fulfill the requirements in the daily work life, as part of the actual breath of its ongoing operations. This is accomplished through an intentional strategic cultural development program.

SEEKING WHAT WE ALREADY HAVE

Not allowing our colleagues an opportunity to discover and explore their strengths means, we are simply choosing to ignore many of the wonderful attributes of our colleagues in our midst. These strengths may lie dormant, unbeknownst to leaders and to the colleague. There is a well-known speech given by Russell Conwell over 6,000 times in early 1900 titled "Acres of Diamonds." Conwell shares in his speech a true story that goes something like this:

Acres of Diamonds

An aged priest told an ancient Persian farmer, Ali Hafed, that if he had a handful of diamonds he could purchase a whole country, and with a mine of diamonds he could place his children upon thrones through the influence of their great wealth. After Al Hafed heard all about diamonds and how much they were worth, he went to his bed that night a poor man — not that he had lost anything, but poor because he was discontented, because he thought he was poor. He said, "I want a mine of diamonds! I want to be immensely rich."

So he decided to leave his farm to seek his fortune. He sold his property, took the proceeds, left his family with neighbors, and set out to seek his fortune. He wandered throughout the region and on into Europe, but never once found the diamonds he was seeking. One day, destitute, disappointed and disheartened, he threw himself into the ocean and finally ended his suffering.

Later, the same priest who told Al Hafed about diamonds came to visit the new property owner and he saw a flash of light from the mantel. He rushed up and said, "Here is a diamond! Here is a diamond! Has Al Hafed returned?" "No, no; Al Hafed has not returned and that is not a diamond. That is nothing but a stone. We found it right out here in our garden." "But I know a diamond when I see it," exclaimed the priest. "That is a diamond!" It did not look like a diamond because it was in its raw, uncut state. In fact, upon closer inspection, they found that the farmland was rich with diamonds. And thus were discovered the diamond mines of Golconda, the most magnificent diamond mines in all the history of mankind.[xxx]

The sad irony of this story is that Ali Hafed wasted his life seeking what he already had in his own backyard. His wealth and fame were right beneath his feet, but he did not recognize diamonds in their raw form. This story holds a wonderful lesson for us. Often, we spend so much time searching "out there in the world" for our happiness, wealth, and significance that we miss many golden opportunities that are right in front of us. In a healthy culture of colleague development, diamonds could already be within our building.

Using the talents and abilities in our current workplace delivers a great opportunity, if we would only ponder the possibilities. Many wonderful opportunities have been lost as we look for "greener" pastures and fail to develop the colleagues we have. But beware, as Erma Bombeck once wrote, "The grass is always greener over the septic tank. I survey the backyard of my life to find that which I am eagerly searching. I look around me with new eyes and a more receptive attitude. I appreciate those situations and conditions in my life that I may have dismissed because I failed to see the good that they hold for me."

See Beyond Position to Uncover Strengths

People are like diamonds in many ways. I realize that not every colleague instantly appears to be a diamond, but maybe we need to look closer at who they are and what their strengths may be. It could be a colleague working in the wrong position for their strengths where they continue to stay in their role for financial security. Discovering a person's strengths is like going on a diamond mining adventure. The diamonds are there. We need to help colleagues discover and recognize their diamond value and help them believe in themselves so they can shine. If we invest in our colleagues and help them to grow personally as well as professionally within our organizations then everyone will get what they want. Investing in our healthcare colleagues will bring greater quality of care for patients, healthy cultures, and greater financial gains for organizations.

Jewels of personal strengths are tremendously valuable on their own merit and allow incredible things to happen spontaneously in organizations. Valuing others brings satisfaction and edification to those that possess them by their illuminations and unique significance. This value of the strength will continuously compound in worth as long as they are treasured and fully appreciated in the organization.

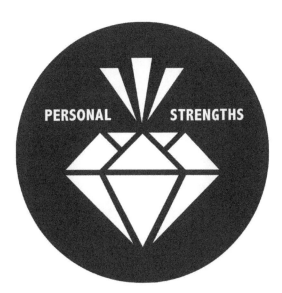

Figure 7

OUR PERSONAL STRENGTHS SYMBOL

The Corporate Transcendence™ Personal Strengths Symbol[xxxii] features a brilliant diamond. When any individual is allowed to work in their strength zone, they shine. When we give out a Personal Strengths icon, we recognize that someone has worked to understand their own strengths and has chosen to use their strengths for the good of the patient, team, or organization. They are truly shining. One beautiful thing about strengths is that you never have to wonder if you've found them. When you are using your strengths, it shows. Any person using their strengths will feel their positive influence grow. Every person in your organization – from the front line to the organizations executives – has unique gifts. Unearthing, polishing, and valuing them will transform your organization

Culture Transformation Action Steps:

Frontline Staff:

Be a strength finder in yourself and in others. Understand, and use your strengths for the collective good for your patient, care team and organization. Minimalizing your inherent strengths is an injustice to yourself and others. Submerge yourself within your strength zone, so you are able to best support your patient and assigned teams in the most efficient and effective way possible. Becoming aware of the unique strengths of the colleagues you work with makes it possible to achieve high reliably teamwork. Choose to build care teams by choosing colleagues in their areas of strengths. By recognizing and appreciating your colleagues' strengths, you encourage them to continue using and engaging their best for the good of the team.

Managerial Leadership:

It is crucial to develop your personal strengths in the areas of leading people. If you are not naturally strong in leadership, dig into learning and improving your abilities. It is important that you continually develop yourself, so you can help develop others. Without the strength for developing people, you will not optimally deliver in your leadership role. View your work with a succession mindset; ask yourself "how can I develop the colleagues under my leadership to become the next generation of leaders?" You will naturally grow as a leader in your organization when your direct reports have personal and professional growth.

Executive Leadership:

When we believe as leaders, that we can be everything to everybody we are mistaken. Being sensitive to this fact and building a circle of expertise is one of the most important aspects of leadership. Create an inner circle for yourself; find a group of colleagues, who you trust to be honest, and get things done with – and WITHOUT – you. Continually develop your own strengths, so you show up filled up and continue to invest in your team. Grow in leadership by developing your strengths.

CHAPTER 9

Equipping: Building People

• • •

"You don't build a business, you build people,
and then people build the business."

ZIG ZIGLAR

DEFINING EQUIPPING

Equipping colleagues begins from the inside out, giving each person the permission and support to grow and develop themselves as human beings. Equipping transcends providing the tangible resources necessary to do work, and reaches colleagues on a personal level. While work cannot be done without these tangible resources, it is equally impossible for our colleagues to perform optimally, and be all they can be without the intentional, ongoing personal equipping process. Not only do we need to be giving people the opportunity to operate in their strengths zones, equipping helps people expand their strengths. It will help them to stretch themselves to be the best they were created to be.

I cannot overemphasize that this is not simply about equipping people to complete a task; equipping is also giving them the freedom and ability to grow and develop themselves as human beings. Without developing our human healthcare assets, we are playing from half a deck. Equipping leaders always ask themselves how to bring the best out of each colleague and how to continue to grow their potential. When we acknowledge the fact that colleagues are our most valuable and appreciable asset, putting focus into equipping them makes sense for the culture, quality, finance, and governance components of the organization. Growing leaders from within through personal equipping creates a strong, vibrant organization, prepares for built-in succession, and returns the highest dividends.

EQUIPPING THE MIND, BODY, AND SOUL

Throughout the course of an eight- or twelve-hour shift, healthcare colleagues perform thousands of mental and physical tasks. It can be physically, emotionally, mentally, and even spiritually draining to fulfill the caregiver role. This must be recognized by leaders in healthcare organizations. The single function of healthcare is taking care of the needs of other people. Each colleague must be equipped with the proper resources and equipment for their work. It would be impossible to function in healthcare without computers, needles, sphygmomanometers, anesthesia units, medications, and others among thousands of tools required daily to care for patients in healthcare organizations.

Think of healthcare caregivers like a person performing in a triathlon. It takes many days of vigorous personal training and preparation to be ready to complete a triathlon. There has to be proper diet, hydration, clothes, but also equipment like shoes, bicycle, headwear, glasses, and water bottles. In addition, and probably most importantly, there must be mental preparation. To prepare and sustain our healthcare teams, we must care for their essential needs, equip them to do the work, and prepare their minds for the rigors of their jobs.

It also takes a great deal of physical, mental, and emotional energy for leadership to do what they must each day, and the same is true for our colleagues. Putting the "human" back in healthcare is not purely about the patient; it certainly needs to be about our colleagues as well. Equipping does not begin just with new tools or competence enhancement training. It begins with caring for your colleagues as human beings and meeting their needs where they are at.

MASLOW'S HIERARCHY OF BASIC HUMAN NEEDS

Abraham Maslow's Hierarchy of Human Needs[xxxiv] established the reasons for this in 1943: we as humans have the same needs. Healthcare is an industry of serving people with basic needs. It is also an industry of people with basic needs taking care of other people with those same needs. Understanding this concept completely is pivotal to properly equipping physically and mentally for an effective healthcare team.

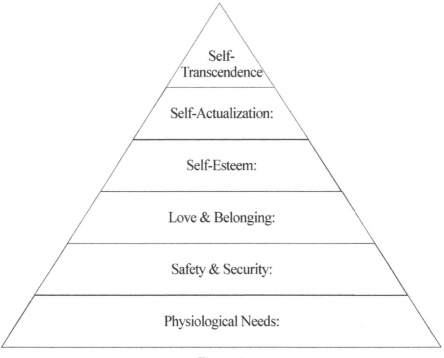

Self-
Transcendence

Self-Actualization:

Self-Esteem:

Love & Belonging:

Safety & Security:

Physiological Needs:

Figure 8

You have likely heard of Maslow's Pyramid starting at its base with physiological needs and building to the top level of self-actualization. Late in Maslow's career, he added an element to the pinnacle, naming it "self-transcendence." He said "The self only finds its actualization in giving itself to some higher goal outside oneself, in altruism and spirituality." Most people who decide to enter a healthcare career do so in order to help and serve others and make a difference in the lives of people. This is a self-transcending activity. In order to operate at that high level, it is necessary for healthcare colleagues to make sure their basic needs are met; otherwise they do not have the capacity to focus and move to the higher levels of self-actualization and transcendence.

CHARACTERISTICS OF BASIC HUMAN NEEDS
1. Needs are universal.
2. Needs may be met in different ways.
3. Needs may be stimulated by external and internal factors.
4. Priorities may be deferred.
5. Needs are interrelated.

Each individual has unique characteristics, but certain needs are common to all people. A need is something that is desirable, useful or necessary. Human needs are physiological and psychological conditions that an individual must meet to achieve a state of health or well-being.

PHYSIOLOGICAL NEEDS:
* Oxygen
* Fluids
* Nutrition
* Elimination
* Rest and sleep
* Sex

Safety and Security Needs:

* Physical safety
* Psychological safety
* Shelter and freedom from harm and danger

Love and Belonging Needs:

* To love and be loved
* To care and to be cared for
* Affection and belonging
* Fruitful and meaningful relationships
* Association with people, institutions, or organizations

Self-Esteem Needs:

* Self-worth
* Self-identity
* Self-respect
* Body image

Self-Actualization Needs

* To learn, create and understand or comprehend
* Harmonious relationships
* Beauty or aesthetics
* Spiritual fulfillment

Characteristics of a Self-Transcendent Person

1. Is realistic, sees life clearly, and is objective about his or her observations
2. Judges people correctly

3. Has superior perception, is more decisive
4. Has a clear notion of right or wrong
5. Is usually accurate in predicting future events
6. Understands art, music, politics, and philosophy
7. Possesses humility, listens to others carefully
8. Is dedicated to some work, task, duty, or vocation
9. Is highly creative, flexible, spontaneous, courageous, and willing to make mistakes
10. Is open to new ideas
11. Is self-confident and has self-respect
12. Has low degree of self-conflict; personality is integrated
13. Does not need fame, and possesses a feeling of self-control
14. Is highly independent, desires privacy
15. Can appear remote or detached
16. Is friendly, loving, and governed more by inner directives than by society
17. Can make decisions contrary to popular opinion
18. Is problem-centered rather than self-centered
19. Accepts the world for what it is

COLLEAGUES ARE HUMANS

The sickness struggles of our patients can take a toll on their family members and the caregivers. Consider this example. An imaging technologist and radiologist may work in a Pediatric department, performing CAT scan images of young children and babies. They observe daily young tender lives affected by or possibly dying from terminal illnesses. In this example, the Imaging Technologist and radiologist is affected emotionally, mentally, physically, and spiritually as a human being. Healthcare workers literally save and change lives daily in our healthcare organizations and they need strong support in all the above ways to be able to give to the patients optimally.

PEOPLE CANNOT GIVE WHAT THEY DO NOT HAVE

We often assume that the equipping process for a healthcare provider solely takes place in their professional schooling. The majority of healthcare workers will share that the equipping they received in school was the technical knowledge preparation to succeed in their new occupation. They were not prepared for the mental, physical and emotional strain, or the exhaustion of the real day-to-day job.

The evidence of this fact is clearly noted by colleagues in our healthcare industry today. People cannot give what they do not have. Healthcare workers cannot be expected to perform their best without the necessary support to grow personally and professionally whether inside or outside the organization. Colleagues focus on what their leaders focus on. The healthcare industry needs to reconsider the employer-employee or organization-colleague relationship. Some healthcare leaders have excelled in this area, but many continue to struggle in the what, when, and how to successfully equip and support their colleagues for organizational success.

Leaders need to create an environment that supports and draws the best qualities from their colleagues. It is an amazing process when you help people discover things about themselves that they may not know. The results are miraculous. The organization has the ability to release the many possibilities of greatness inside every colleague, which will result in a better-equipped caregiver functioning daily in the organization.

CREATE A TRANSFORMATIONAL ENVIRONMENT

The secret to sustained organizational success in mastering a transformational environment of excellence begins first and foremost with transforming individuals. In personal transformation, leaders set the example. Leaders transform first, and work to discover and understand their own strengths through continued personal and professional development. This allows leaders to build good relationships with colleagues. This improved connection enables leaders to influence colleagues in embracing the mission, vision, and needs of the organization. Then colleagues follow and press forward to positively propel the organization to continued improvement and excellence.

Leaders and their colleagues should be seen as masterpieces being shaped for improving themselves all the time. Many times we lose sight of this fact. Unconsciously, we often assume that people have already achieved their maximum potential. If they are not great at something – or perfect in some role – we assume there is something wrong with them. Rather than looking for areas where they need equipping to expand their capacity, we throw them off the bus and start looking for a new person to meet our need. Colleagues who consistently perform well can be judged and be seen differently as soon as they make a mistake. Human beings seem to naturally remember the bad instead of the good in people. That is why we do not need to view others or ourselves as being perfect. We all make mistakes and foul up at times. But if we look at mistakes as just that, and learn from them and become more equipped due to what we learn through the mistakes we are making, this is called "failing forward." This naming practice helps to resolve negative feelings about oneself and towards others.

Perhaps we should acknowledge the pervasive negativity that is all around us. Continuous, negative news flows from our media, imputing negative feelings into our environments. The power of this negativity, without the balance of positivity, is dangerous to the well-being of others, and to our society. But rather than internalizing the negativity and letting it filter what we see in our work, we can remember that humans are humans and, as humans, all will make mistakes. Healthcare workers do not invest big slices of their lives and finances in educational institutions with the intention of making a poor decision for the patients they prepared so long and hard to help.

How mistakes are handled by an individual, and how people accepts this, tells others of what character of people or leaders we are. When someone makes an unintentional mistake, we need to rewire our minds and consider with understanding what we could do to help support the colleague, and keep it from reoccurring. All colleagues need an environment that supports self-reflection and education as needed so future errors are not repeated. An environment that allows colleagues a voice and personal, professional development is an environment that stimulates proactive thinking to reduce errors or mistakes.

A toxic environment develops when leaders set the example of fear and retaliation for mistakes. Colleagues will align their actions to survive in this environment. It is obvious when colleagues do not support this type of social work life environment. It will be palpable and well known by all colleagues. This culture is verbally shared in the water cooler communication of the organization.

Rather than fixate on the negative, encourage your employees to grow by allowing them to explore and better understand their own seeds of greatness. The fostered individual strengths will develop and create the "secret sauce" that makes an organization soar to heights never before imagined. This requires a safe environment that will draw out improvements and the greatness in their employees. Most employees, when given the opportunities for growth, will transform to become a more valuable employee in the organization.

Culture that dives deep into the talents of colleagues will discover many gems. Do not judge the job title or the surface appearance. Consider that a colleague who punches in and out each day with minimal professional education may be one of the brightest gems in your organization. This colleague may just need to receive some coaching and development to understand the greatness that is already uniquely theirs. Healthcare colleagues are the core of the organization. The better-equipped the colleagues are, the stronger the core of the organization will be.

People Are the Core

Remember, our colleagues are the central core of the organization and not the periphery. If we treat them like they are on the fringes on our organization, they will perform more as supporting actors than the leading stars. They are the stars in healthcare. Colleagues will win the day in people's lives every single day, if equipped and empowered properly for personal and professional success.

It takes money, time, and energy to support colleagues. There is a vast reservoir of personal strengths that colleagues bring to the table, as we discussed in Chapter 8, Personal Strengths: Cultivating High Performance. Tapping into these strengths is an economical way to bring value to the colleagues and provide personal development to them. Many frontline colleagues enjoy teaching and would be useful in leading personal growth workshops to peers. Consider the employees who are excellent role models employees; they would be awesome to teach the importance of core values and how they play into an organization's core values. Perhaps this group of colleagues could be empowered to help leadership develop core values for the organization.

CREATE A LEARNING ENVIRONMENT

The best learning environment for colleagues is created when the teachers and trainers largely originate from within the organization. To have the necessarily robust educational curriculum within the organization, it does not require tens or hundreds of thousands of dollars to be paid annually to outside coaches, trainers, and consultants on an ongoing basis. In the beginning, it may require coaching, often external training, and mentoring to the organization's leaders and colleagues to get started on this path to excellence, but it is critical to ongoing success for the organization to customize its own talent and its own best practices. Creating a learning environment and change a culture will take leadership intentionality.

In determining how to equip the colleagues to obtain the most value for the organization, it is not teaching of policy, procedures, or how to perform a particular task better that will make the greatest impact on the development of a high reliability organization. Although these things are important and required, the greatest impact is when colleagues receive personal development that improves their lives on a deeper more meaningful level. This type of equipping brings the greatest dedication and commitment to excellence from colleagues.

Engaging colleagues to learn is vital in order to perform optimally in their duties. They constantly need to receive training and education to prevent errors. As human beings, we naturally desire to enrich and expand our lives in many ways. Providing opportunities for colleagues to explore areas of personal growth is self-edifying and provides a sense of self-worth and esteem. Personal development opens the mind to new and creative ideas that can greatly benefit an organization to achieving success and becoming its best. A few examples of personal development topics that could be shared in a workshop or a Mastermind group would be:

- Public speaking (Yes you CAN)
- Personal and organization core values
- How to facilitate a meeting effectively
- Discovering and valuing personal strengths
- What the value of empathy
- How to successfully build a the DREAM team
- Customizing the process improvement model
- Developing the leader in me

The list of possible topics cannot be exhausted. All topics can directly and indirectly enhance the colleague's performance and contributions to the organization, as well as to the colleague's personal life. This is a double win for the colleague, resulting in a happier and more satisfying life for the people who make up the core of the organization and who ultimately provide the most meaningful contributions to the organization's success. It is rooted inside of each colleague within the organization. If an organization wants to be great, they start with equipping their colleagues for greatness and positive effects. Below is a listing of a few of the positive benefits from equipping colleagues:

Positive Benefits of Colleague Equipping

* Equipping builds excellence.
* Equipping invests in the future.
* Equipping engages the colleague.
* Equipping breathes success into the organization.
* Equipping makes the difference in the delivery of healthcare.
* Equipping saves and changes lives not only for colleagues, but for patients

Equipping Matters

Equip the colleague to enjoy better quality of health by providing a wellness program for them. Equip the colleague to be vocal. Give them a voice to express thoughts, suggestions, and ideas. Self-expression is an essential aspect of human life. Equip the colleagues to be heard. Emphasize the importance of respecting and valuing each voice. Equip colleagues with everything they need. Make all the boundaries clear, and they will be able to respect them. Show colleagues they are valued and appreciated. Provide an incredible team environment. Expect world-class leadership to be developed in willing managers and leaders. Provide coaching and education for mistakes to allow them to move forward. Give colleagues a nurturing environment so they can give care, compassion, and empathy to their patients. Equip colleagues to be the best person they can be. All people naturally desire to grow and expand their lives.

It is important that colleagues show joy and peace in their tone of voice and the smiles they give away each day. Colleagues do not need to come to work to worry about work. Peace is important. Colleagues are just like all people, they are faced with many challenges in life. Treat colleagues with value and respect, and they will treat others with respect and value.

Figure 9

Our Equipping Symbol

The Corporate Transcendence™ Equipping Symbol[xxxvi] is a single warrior's helmet. This represents the need to equip each person in the organization as an individual. In healthcare, it can often feel like we are heading out to do battle each day. Effectively equipping ourselves and our colleagues protects against the injuries and energy drain that occur without it. Much like a helmet, equipping is something that each colleague must choose to wear. Being fully equipped for excellence requires action on the part of leadership as well as the individual being equipped. Recognition will come naturally for leaders who equip their colleagues as well as colleagues who do the important work of equipping themselves to be the best they can be.

CULTURE TRANSFORMATION ACTION STEPS:

FRONTLINE STAFF:

Accept responsibility for equipping your mind, body, and soul. Search for opportunities to learn and grow in your professional knowledge and in ways to become an improved YOU. Take initiative to be resourced so you can deliver your best. You cannot give what you do not have. People performing at the top "of their game" make the necessary and timely preparation to equip themselves for any task or potential challenge. Continually enhance your abilities and equip your mind to be used in more positive ways.

MANAGERIAL LEADERSHIP:

You should always be on a personal learning journey to continually equip yourself as a manager. Set the example among colleagues for self-equipping through learning opportunities. Be sensitive to potential opportunities daily to support colleagues in improvement of their processes and procedures. You are responsible to make sure your staff has what they need to be most successful in tangible and non-tangible ways. Develop the skills to "manage up" to let the people over you know when things are needed and help your people receive what they need.

EXECUTIVE LEADERSHIP:

Equip your organization first by making sure you have "the right people, in the right seat, on the right bus." You are responsible for the 5 W's (when, why, who, what, and where) for success of your organization. People are your best arsenal for success. Equipping the organization is a making sure all colleagues and areas of operations have every resource that is necessary to be successful.

CHAPTER 10

Empowerment: Releasing Excellence

• • •

"As we look ahead into the next century, leaders will be those who empower others."

BILL GATES

DEFINING EMPOWERMENT

Empowerment is the act of sharing power and giving freedom to unleash the talents and strengths of the people who work in your organization. Empowerment encourages them to do their best and to know they are in a safe space to use their gifts. Empowerment encourages colleagues to work harder, do more, and achieve best outcomes. Empowerment leaves no room for micromanaging, rather involves creating teams and allowing them to thrive. Empowerment allows people to engage their own personal drive and unique gifts to accomplish the goal and daily tasks in front of them. Organizations that have achieved a high reliability level will be empowering, and because of that, the organization's mission will live and breathe throughout day-to-day operations.

This type of functionality brings a common purpose and direction to the organization that is not mandated from higher leadership staff, but driven mostly from other colleagues. Empowerment is also a strategic strengthening strategy that increases your influence and effectiveness as a leader. Releasing people to do what they are great at inspires them to bring the best of their strengths and attitude to your organization. Limiting empowerment to colleagues from the top" provides microscopic gains compared to drastic improvement that comes from unleashing people at every level. Empowerment goes beyond decision-making. It edifies the identity and self-image of someone's place in the organization.

Unleashing the Power

Empowerment is the ultimate releasing of the greatest power of the organization. We must release the power in order to progress the organization to excellence or beyond. Earlier chapters discuss how and why it is important to connect and positively influence colleagues, but unless you truly release colleagues in a culture of personal and professional growth; the culture will be sick and even die. It would be like keeping a butterfly jailed in a cocoon when it has transformed into an amazing beautiful creation. Not only is it a waste of the beautiful wings, it is a new strength and ability to fly will be lost as the constraints eventually kill it.

Empowerment must have a giver and a receiver. There must be an individual giving their authority or power to another person in order for them to use their own authority or power in situations or experiences. An example is the first time you allow your child to cash out a purchase alone in a grocery store. The child is empowered by the parent to purchase out the item from the cashier and to count out the correct amount of money to pay for the item. The empowerment allows the child to develop and learn.

Adults just like children must be able to continually grow as individuals. This is a need in all humans. When empowered, colleagues must be allowed to test their wings, and eventually understand how to spread their own wings of power and soar. The goal is to develop colleagues who are comfortable in their own so called feathers of greatness and make sure they experience the appreciation of their work as it adds value of the organization.

Leadership giving colleagues empowerment is a staging process when taking an organization from average to excellence and beyond. Colleague empowerment will be one of the most valuable tools for establishing systematic, sustainable excellence in an organization. In fact, it will be the fuel that drives the perpetual success in the organization. Never underestimate its worth or its power. Colleague connected and empowered with an organization who are allowed to use their influence in every way imaginable will not only take an organization to excellence but can lead it to transcendence. There will be no limit, no walls, no barriers to the excellence achieved when compounded talents and strengths of the colleagues are released.

Colleagues that engage will many times surprise themselves as well as leadership, in their creativity, innovation, and excellence in ideas, thoughts, and actions within the organization.

Empowerment Characteristics

Below are examples of outcomes observed as the result of colleagues being empowered in an organization? These observations allow a more in-depth look at empowerment as a cause and effect in an organization. Empowerment of colleagues is key to achieving excellence and creating a transcendent organization as demonstrated below in these examples.

* Intoxicating and invigorating.
* Builds energy and momentum.
* Elevates the cognitive ability of an organization through connectivity of ideas.
* Develops trust – people giving power away to others.
* Invests in other people's abilities.
* Motivates people to take action.
* Develops skills and abilities.
* Builds morale.
* Contagious in the workplace.

CREATING AN EMPOWERING ENVIRONMENT

Empowerment is not pixie dust that can be sprinkled on colleagues, magically bestowing the skills needed to perform certain task with authority and confidence. Empowerment can be nurtured or killed at any time. The culture in your organization needs specific elements in order to foster empowerment. Empowerment is the product of a well-defined corporate systemic initiative and supported by a well-designed infrastructure. Education is a major factor for colleagues to be successfully empowered. Leaders need to build the confidence and competence of each colleague by providing feedback in private and complementing in public. In order for colleagues to rise up and embrace their empowered status, they must feel safe from fear and intimidation. This is why a culture of trust is necessary if colleagues are to be effectively empowered.

Empowerment has an edifying factor. It instills intellectual credibility. It lifts people up and increases job satisfaction, boosting morale when colleagues know that others believe in them.

ONLY LEADERS EMPOWER

Theodore Roosevelt is reported as saying "The best executive is one who has sense enough to pick good people to do what he wants done, and self-restraint enough to keep from meddling with them while they do it." Imagine what we could accomplish in healthcare if we could create this kind of empowerment on our teams? General George Smith Patton, Jr. said "Never tell people how to do things. Tell them what to do and they will surprise you with their ingenuity."

Promoting and supporting empowerment in an organization conveys a lot about its leaders. You will not have insecure leaders advocating empowerment. Empowering leaders will be leaders who are comfortable in their own skin. They are not afraid of giving up power others – in fact they relish the thought. They give others the opportunity to develop and gain power as much as possible.

Controlling, low self-esteem and micromanaging leaders will be conflicted in an empowering environment. If empowerment is difficult for you, reflect on what controlling insecurities and micromanaging habits may have developed in your map of the world.

EMPOWERMENT AT VARIOUS LEVELS

Empowering leaders understand the scales of balanced power. The power is distributed and balanced according to the skills and abilities of the colleagues. Take this story as an example.

A patient registration colleague in a hospital is checking in a patient to have an diagnostic imaging procedure performed, but due to an unexpected emergency with another patient, the scheduled patient is delayed an hour beyond their appointment time. The patient is upset, the delay affecting his return to work as planned that day. Instead of the registration colleague ignoring his frustration, the colleague is empowered to conduct service recovery. The patient registration colleague apologizes and offer the patient some coffee, and to reschedule their appointment to a more convenient time and day, or to give a free lunch voucher for the hospital cafeteria. The colleagues are empowered to take action that demonstrates empathy and values the patient from their point of view. The patient satisfaction may be salvageable by this empowered colleague. Without empowerment, the patient registration colleague may offer a feeble "we apologize for the inconvenience." The hospitality industry has used similar service recovery techniques for years. For example, Marriott has a policy that allows colleagues to spend up to a certain amount of money to satisfy a guest.

Patients who choose our healthcare organization are our guests. Performing service recovery is an example of empathy and empowerment working hand in hand. This echoes the *platinum rule:* "doing unto others" as they would like for you to do unto them.

Unbalanced Empowerment

Unbalanced empowerment comes when leadership is asking a colleague to perform a task for which they possess neither the training nor the competency to perform successfully. Based on the above example if the patient registration staff had not adequate training in service recovery it may lead to a disastrous outcome. In a situation, where a patient may raise their voice and speak rudely to the registration staff, the empowered colleague should know clearly from corporate training what they should do.

Balanced Empowerment

Balanced empowerment is also allowing frontline colleagues a voice in the organization by involving them on teams and committees. This allows them to provide a frontline perspective and approach to problem solving.

Listening as a leader to colleagues can be an empowering experience for the colleagues. Lunch meetings between leadership and colleagues will provide great insight for leadership, and also give colleagues a venue to have a voice and share ideas that are valuable.

Leadership that supports empowerment constantly seeks opportunities to use the talents and strengths of their colleagues throughout the organization more. Tapping into and empowering the use of these strengths builds positive momentum and creates a top performing organization. This communicates across the organization that success of empowered colleagues creates greater success for the organization. Some of the payoffs for all colleagues and the organization as a whole are listed below:

What Empowerment Creates

* Fosters ownership
* Motivates colleagues

* Builds self-worth
* Encourages ingenuity
* Stretches colleagues outside their comfort zone
* Supports teamwork
* Solves problems
* Recognizes gifts and skills
* Fulfills and rewards colleagues
* Allows for personal expression
* Improves colleague morale
* Fosters colleague engagement
* Builds competence
* Supports a learning environment
* Maximizes efficiency.
* Amplifies positive momentum.
* Allows leadership to flourish at level.
* Bonds connection to mission, vision and core values of organization.
* Propels collaborative movement toward lasting success.

Creating and fostering a culture that is healthy is essential to having an environment that will stimulate individuals to engage in the empowerment process. In a healthy culture, colleagues will use this empowerment authority for the greater good of the organization.

This is the difference in a colleague declaring "I don't mind working" and "I love my job. I look forward to going to work."

People Feel Valued

When we choose to empower colleagues, it says that they as individuals matter, their thoughts matter, their work matters, their extra efforts matter. It gives them the understanding that they make the organization more successful because of their empowerment.

People Feel Ownership:

When colleagues are empowered they have a sense of ownership in the organization beyond their normal work activities. They feel responsible and accountable for what they are doing and how it will affect others. They have a stake in the game so to speak, and are more conscious of the impact they can and do have on the organization as a whole.

Colleagues desire success in their organization and themselves as the outcome of their efforts. When they use the freedom empowerment gives them to act, and get a good result; it demonstrates that their choice makes a positive difference. They will feel a sense of accomplishment.

Inspired to Leverage Empowerment

Empowerment is an amazing characteristic to witness in a colleague. I am always amazed at its energy, power, and the positive momentum it can build in an organization. If colleagues feel empowered they will create, develop, and help build organizational excellence.

Empowerment unlocks the individual potential of a person and releases abilities that many times others were not aware that they possessed. The individual sometimes may not know they possess the abilities, because no one ever gave them an open door to use them.

With empowerment, I have seen colleagues work harder and sacrifice greater to achieve best results in situations. If colleagues are to continue bringing their best efforts, they must know that their efforts will be celebrated and recognized. Most of all, they must be the ones who receive the accolades for their appropriate use of power. Empowerment of colleagues is about them and their work and success, not leadership or management.

Empowerment has to be a developmental process, built upon trust. Personal and professional colleague development allows an organization to discover the strengths and talents of their colleagues. This naturally leads to colleagues having opportunities to use their strengths. Colleagues also must be engaged to become empowered. Colleague engagement is the critical link to empowerment. Without engagement there will not be empowerment.

EMPOWERMENT INCREASES EXPERTISE

An example of empowerment would be allowing a group of colleagues to plan and implement a colleague Appreciation Day. There is a great chance for the event it to turn out wonderfully, allowing the colleagues to feel valued and trusted for being an integral part of the celebration.

Empowerment is also letting those that do a particular job or function have a say in how it can be improved or if it should be revised or changed. It is true if you want to know how to improve something you ask the individuals that do that job. We need to consider them as the expert.

If we are sick, we go to a doctor, thinking that a person who practices medicine will have the greater knowledge and understanding of the illness. If we want to have a beautifully landscaped yard, we need to seek expert advice from a gardener or a landscaper to get the look we desire. People who study an area or repeatedly work in a certain area of expertise will always be able to provide greater insight.

The problem I have observed when empowering colleagues is that leaders and managers get in the way or suppress the empowerment. As leaders and managers, we often feel that we know better or can do something better due to our experience or our knowledge. The truth is, many times this is not the case. In spite of our vast wisdom, education, and experience; frontline colleagues will have more pertinent information when it comes to optimal patient care.

As I have built empowering cultures for colleagues working in healthcare at all levels of the organization, a focus has been to remove myself or be sensitive to not get in their way. Releasing the colleagues to successfully accomplish work in their personal way will make the organization stronger.

This highly effective, frontline approach is often overlooked. When there is a new requirement to be addressed in healthcare, many times the people who do the job related to the requirement are not involved in the decision making in how to meet the new requirement. This creates more confusion and does not build engagement or empowerment.

To build a core of excellence, all people matter and their thoughts hold value. Leaders have to believe this and act accordingly. Bringing in the missing voices will bring all the pieces of the puzzle so to speak to the table. When leading meetings, it is important to insure all people directly and indirectly related to the topic of the meeting are present. Meetings like this declare that all voices are heard, all thoughts are valued, all people matter.

This message must be repeated by leadership, management and all of the colleagues. It must be a fundamental belief of the organization, not just in theory but in practice and application. An organization can describe this message using the metaphor of each colleague being the CEO of their role and environment.

Imagine a work environment in a hospital where each colleague – regardless of their title or their work – is told they are all considered to be Chiefs in their areas. They have ownership in its success and their contribution is seen as highly valued and important. This is horizontal organizational infrastructure where empowerment is instilled in every colleague.

Can you imagine the power of this mindset? The momentum – the success – that would be continuously building? Empowered colleagues may be so excited about their work that it feels more like play than work at times. Empowerment is edifying.

You may be thinking that this is a pipe dream and not possible, but the good news is it is possible and achievable. You can see this "dream" walking your halls every day if you desire.

Empowerment can only be brought out in individuals that do not harbor fear. Many times the colleague has to step out of a comfort zone to exercise empowerment. Empowerment is not a dominating behavior. Empowerment brings more accountability and responsibility to colleagues. It is a shared power for the betterment and good of others and the organization as a whole. To better clarify the meaning of empowerment, let look at what is NOT empowerment.

EMPOWERMENT IS NOT:

* Empowerment is not entitlement.
* Empowerment is not self-serving.
* Empowerment is not about ego.
* Empowerment is not selfish.
* Empowerment does not retaliate.

Empowerment may need to have some boundaries, but the boundaries should not create feelings of entrapment in that the colleague cannot function independently in the decision making that is needed.

A mouse may be released to run through a maze, but if the mouse continues to run into a dead end, he may stop trying to exercise his empowerment to run and just stop trying. Just like this example, colleagues who get hedged in by fear or lose hope will lose the confidence that is needed to feel empowered.

Below is a list of barriers that limit colleagues from enjoying empowerment in their work. A culture of healing works to eliminate these barriers.

EMPOWERMENT BARRIERS

* Lip service of shared power by leaders without action.
* Insecure leaders that must retain control.
* Inconsistency in empowerment release.
* Micromanagement of empowered colleagues.
* Lack of trust among leaders and colleagues.
* Misleading on poorly-defined boundaries.

* Undermining a decision or second guessing.
* Inadequate training for empowerment of duties and tasks.

From these barriers it is easy to see that open transparent and highly communicable environment is important in having colleague engagement and empowerment. It is absolutely amazing to see and experience the result from true empowerment in actions among colleagues. Colleague empowerment is worth the investment of education and resources, and is a true mark of a more successful and sophisticated culture of excellence.

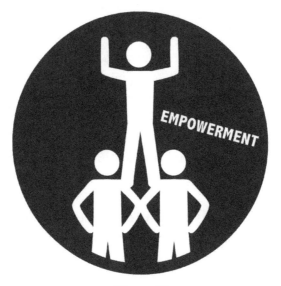

Figure 10

Our Empowerment Symbol

The Corporate Transcendence™ Empowerment Symbol[xxxviii] depicts the process of sharing power among colleagues. Together, leaders form the base for empowering individuals to rise to the top of their ability. We recognize the value of empowerment at every level of the organization. Any time two people work together; there is the potential to share power with one another in order to maximize the strengths of each person.

Culture Transformation Action Steps:

Frontline Staff:

As a frontline colleague, you have to believe in yourself and be comfortable in your own skin. Recognize through an empowering culture, your organization believes in your talents and what you have to contribute. When you have the opportunity to exercise your skills and strengths, jump in! Being empowered allows you to impact your environment, regardless of your role. Tap into your sense of ownership which feeds your empowerment, and do your part to make the environment an excellent one for your colleagues and patients.

Managerial Leadership:

You have to first believe in your frontline colleagues. Give your front line the space to stretch their empowerment capacity. If you are struggling with this, dig back into the practice of valuing; recognize and affirm your staff and their strengths. Everyone has the internal desire to be more and do more. Give them space to shine. Empower them effectively and they will be motivated to do more than what is expected.

Executive Leadership:

Because each person on the team has an individual area of expertise, you need to create an open, welcoming environment of good intentions so that everyone feels they can bring their best and honest thoughts forward. The stakes are high in the executive leadership circle. Passion and cordial disagreements are necessary and healthy to discussions at this level. All leadership comes to a consensus, so that everyone walks away from the meeting with harmony. Executives foster empowerment for colleagues at every level, and in every department throughout the organization.

CHAPTER 11

Momentum:
Collective Energy Force

• • •

*"The amount of effort needed at the start pales in comparison
to what your momentum can ultimately produce in the end."*

LINCOLN PATZ

DEFINING MOMENTUM

Positive momentum in an organization is the collective energy force of
individuals that propels every aspect of an organization as it evolves to
excellence and beyond. Positive Momentum occurs when any machine is
running well, when all movement is going in the right direction for best
results. Momentum makes it possible for our excellence tomorrow to always be better than our excellence today. Momentum is generated within
the people of an organization, produced from their ongoing development
inside of a healthy culture. You do not get positive organizational momentum out of physical structure – it comes from within people.

THE POWER OF MOMENTUM

As a world-record breaker and a six-time gold medalist, Usain Bolt from
Jamaica knows a thing or two about momentum. The star athlete casts a

powerful model for running hopefuls that is alluringly transferrable to the healthcare field. Although many would declare his own track antics as partly "insane," there is no denying the pure power and speed of this man. He has awesome positive mental and physical momentum!

What if our healthcare organizations had a small slice of the momentum that the "lightning bolt" has? What if we had a clear direction, and moved swiftly towards our goals with the same intense internal urgency and passion? Just as Usain Bolt must understand all the part of his physical being to be able to win gold medals, also we must understand the effect our momentum has on an organization.

I describe an organization as a living, breathing organism made up of unique individuals working toward common goals. There is no question that organizations can possess oscillating energy levels, similar to the stock market fluctuation. Organization organisms possess different levels of energy, motion and emotions, just by the simple fact they consist of human beings and human beings are unique unto themselves. Understanding and remembering this fact will be essential to providing effective leadership, maximizing success, and fueling momentum in an organization.

Momentum in Healthcare

Working in an organization that has high momentum can be incredibly satisfying. There is an atmosphere of positive adrenalin, energy, excitement, and enthusiasm. The greater the force, energy, and drive the more positive the results in organizations. Just as surfers wait anxiously for a monumental wave of strength, called the "Big Mo" wave, to catch an awesome experience riding their surfboards, leaders look for that push of energy and accomplishment to move their colleagues forward. The higher momentum environment builds anticipation and frequent "wins" which are observed and felt by colleagues. Winning creates opportunities for celebration, produces happy feelings, and positively reinforces behavior that promotes the "Big Mo" to continually build and sustain itself.

There have been a number of research studies completed that back up the effects of positive momentum. An interesting study on the effect on positive feelings to negative feelings relate to a study by Dr. Barbara Frederickson of the University of North Carolina. Dr. Frederickson, a prominent scientist concluded that in the study of positive emotions, humans need a positive ratio of 3:1. We need three positive emotions to balance every one negative emotion if we are to reap the benefit of the positive feeling.[xxxix]

In another study, Dr. Marcial Losada dealt with human capital and team effectiveness, demonstrating that the highest performing teams have a positive ratio of 6:1. Positive experiences and high momentum are essential in an organization to achieve peak effectiveness.[xl] Both studies reveal achieving positive momentum and results requires effort.

There are many benefits to momentum that go beyond its advantage in accomplishing organizational goals. Momentum is tied to sustainable success and an organization's reputation for leading in its industry. Top healthcare organizations possess high momentum are never satisfied. Creating high positive momentum in healthcare organizations require an intentional, ongoing focused initiative by its leaders. It requires leadership that provides systemic, strategic efforts, in order to generate ongoing positive momentum from internal planning.

Momentum is a common term often used in sports announcements, describing a team that is taking positive action to win games. These actions result in overcoming the competition. Fortune 500 companies have realized the importance of momentum and invest heavily in training and incentives to create the positive energy around selling products and services. The bottom line? Momentum matters.

Assessing Momentum

Organizations as a whole can possess different levels of momentum over a period of time. Sometimes momentum can differ from one department to another from one nursing floor to another. Let's discuss the many different levels of momentum. High, medium, low, or nominal energy momentum levels could all exist in an organization. An organization can also be described as a status quo organization where forward momentum is totally lacking. The goal in any organization is to have the positive momentum level as high as possible. There are many benefits to high momentum in an organization that definitely are worth the effort.

You may want to take a moment to examine the momentum in your organization. Would you describe your organization as possessing high, medium, low momentum, or would the term status quo best describe your organization?

What level of momentum would you like to have in your organization? Let's examine the various levels of momentum that may be experienced in a healthcare organization.

High Momentum

High momentum is associated with organizations that are successful, often referred to as forward-thinking, up-to-date, or cutting-edge. Many times they are publicly perceived as market leaders among competitors or in the community, state, nation, or world. A high level of momentum is the ideal environment that fosters success and higher colleague's satisfaction. High momentum flows within an infrastructure that allows it to continuously develop colleagues in an organization. High momentum is associated with an organization that has an energetically positive work climate, made up of highly engaged colleagues with high morale. Highly engaged colleagues constantly deliver their best. The colleagues propel the organization forward in a successful rhythm. Positive energy vibrates among the employees.

When you have positive momentum, there is a palpable atmosphere of expectation and enthusiasm that runs through the organization. Team members feel a spirit of excitement and fulfillment in the work being accomplished. When colleagues are asked to describe their organization's energy, they may use words like: enjoyable place to work, a lot of team spirit, progressive, growing, successful, happy, and fulfillment, and the list continues. Having high momentum does not mean colleagues work harder, but it does mean they work smarter and feel good about their work and work culture.

High momentum organizations may sometimes experience a slight dip in their peak momentum level when going through seasons of strategic planning, organizational change, or new goals establishment. Leaders need to be aware of this natural dip. Leaders should always remember that the highest level of momentum possible should be maintained at all times regardless of what is taking place in the organization. The effect of actions by people on the organizational momentum should always be taken into consideration or when major change is strategized. A slight drop in momentum should occur in a shortest period of time possible and as a process for realignment of the organization's new goals to the organization's mission.

There should be an overlap of work activities while realignment or introductions of new goals are implemented. A stall in time between perspective work elements can bring momentum down. Keeping activities ongoing, aligning or adjusting is better than bringing one project to a complete closure before starting another. Leaders must plan and consider ways that momentum is maintained during this period of transition. Supporting this could be celebrating momentum wins in the organization in a spontaneous manner.

It is important to grasp that creating, developing, and maintaining momentum does not occur by accident. When a company gains national recognition as a great place to work, there is a natural expectation that positive things are happening and the organization has a high momentum environment. A high momentum state is intentionally created and maintained by leadership. There is no magic wand or a single silver bullet to create high momentum in an organization. Momentum comes only from intentional design. Achieving and sustaining it requires planning, cultivation, and continuous effort on behalf of the leadership.

CHARACTERISTICS OF HIGH MOMENTUM IN AN ORGANIZATION

Would your organization register a high positive momentum? Below are some indicators that might suggest that your organization is experiencing high momentum:

- Colleagues are highly engaged.
- Colleagues are highly motivated.
- Team spirit leads to collective effectiveness.
- Positive attitudes predominate.
- Innovation and creativity flourish from non-management to leadership.
- Colleagues enjoy a sense of fulfillment from their daily work.
- Every person in the organization has clarity on the mission, vision, and core values.
- Enthusiasm is shared by all.
- Team members experience trusting and respectful relationships.
- Individual strengths and differences are consistently valued.
- Empathy toward colleagues and patients is the standard practice.
- Empowered colleagues lead themselves and their environments.
- The culture is marked by an attitude of service and hospitality.

MEDIUM MOMENTUM

An organization that has medium momentum usually experiences a flux or swing in the momentum range from high to low. This condition represents a weaker infrastructure that prevents sustainability of the momentum at a high level. An analogy of medium or average momentum would be sitting on the beach and watching the various sizes of waves rolling onto the shore line. This could describe medium momentum, as being the average of all the wave sizes or energies.

This is not the lowest level to exist at in the work culture, but certainly not the optimal place for an organization that wants to be at the top of its game or in the coveted top 5% of healthcare organizations. In the medium momentum level, colleagues and department engagement fluctuates, causing some processes and daily functions to have some inherent organizational inconsistencies. The great news it is much easier to reach a consistent high momentum level coming from the medium level versus coming from a lower level. In my experience, it takes minimal tweaking and recalibration in performance areas by leaders to optimize the organization to the highest momentum desired.

Characteristics of Moderate Momentum
If you are experiencing a moderate amount of momentum, you may see these indicators:

* Some colleagues are engaged and others are not.
* Some teams are more effective and successful than others.
* Job satisfaction varies among colleagues.
* Empowerment is limited to a few colleagues.
* Motivation varies among colleagues.
* Both positive and negative attitudes and behaviors exist.
* Empathy, value and respect are not consistently felt among all colleagues.
* Innovation and creativity is sporadic and not spontaneous.
* Understanding of the mission and vision and core values is inconsistent.
* Enthusiasm flows through the individual colleague rather than being shared among groups and teams.

Low Momentum
A place of low momentum is a dangerous level for healthcare organizations to exist. Look for flashing warning signs throughout the organization. Many times communication in the organization is minimal or nonexistent, yielding mistrust. Colleagues feel devalued as workers or

possibly even as human beings. There is unsettledness. Apathy can set in among colleagues. Colleagues that have higher dissatisfaction levels that will overflow into lower patient satisfaction scores. Colleagues will not perform their best if there is major dissatisfaction in the existing work culture. Dissatisfaction becomes a distraction that is concerning due to the lack of or low momentum and undermines the paramount purpose of healthcare, which is the patient.

Low momentum among colleagues should first be addressed from a leadership's perspective. Momentum is a designed strategic initiative from senior leadership, middle management, or a combination of both. Usually there are evident facts for the low momentum that need to be addressed sooner rather than later. The longer the organization stays at this level, the more vulnerable and at risk the organization will become. In a low momentum state, leadership needs to act quickly to get the organization's momentum to a higher level. Low momentum is the most challenging leadership environment to work in. This environment takes a lot more energy and effort to get daily, normal routine work accomplished.

CHARACTERISTICS OF LOW MOMENTUM

If you are experiencing low momentum in your organizations, here are some of the possible signs to be aware of.

* Reduced productivity
* Depressed morale
* Disengaged colleagues
* Low momentum or momentum deficit disorder
* Organization digressing or going in the wrong direction
* Poor or lack of leadership
* Financial concerns
* Trust issues
* Lack of communication
* Low colleague engagement

- Overall colleague dissatisfaction
- Toxic work environment
- High turnover

MOMENTUM TRANSITION

Leaders must become cognizant of the fact that it will take time to bring the organization to a higher momentum state. Processes and systems will need attention to convert the environment from a reactive state into a proactive one. Extra care should also be taken to ensure that the environment does not resemble a roller-coaster amusement ride, moving from low to high, and back again. Low momentum is incredibly stressful for colleagues. A silo mentality among colleagues and the feeling that everyone is looking out for himself is a common survival technique. Leaders must consistently build higher momentum that will require thoughtful planning and collaborations across the organization. Remember, momentum flows from inside of the people through the intentional design of an organization's infrastructure. Develop your colleagues and continually tune the infrastructure for steady improvements and sustainability.

THE STATUS QUO LEDGE

My slogan for "Status Quo" is "Do Not Go!" This is not where we want to lead any organization. Status quo is a place of nominal colleague engagement, insignificant results. Nominal colleague engagement produces a culture of going through the motion of work, void of momentum. This is a dead-end road for organizations. Staying on this road could easily result in the risk of the healthcare organization going out of business. It is like being asleep at the wheel of an automobile, and suddenly you open your eyes and you are upside down in the middle of the road with trucks mowing over you and cars careening around you. I have seen organizations sink to this level and the result is a sick culture organization.

In today's healthcare climate, successful organizations do not have the luxury of remaining unchanged. Status quo will mean death. It only takes a fairly short period of time, like a few months to a few years to fall behind expected industry standards. An example would be a healthcare company not implementing electronic health records in the age of information technology or collecting patient clinical data in regard to federal mandates from legislative healthcare reform. Momentum is part of leadership's responsibility and will affect all aspects of an organization.

Characteristics of the Status Quo Ledge

Status quo permeates an organization going through the motions of the day-to-day, by simply existing. Status quo or negative momentum is problematic, resulting in low colleague motivation. In other words, the organization is stuck in a rut. It is ludicrous to keep doing the same thing over and over again and expecting different results – and that's exactly what the status quo gives us. Status quo also reminds me of a mud puddle that has stagnant water and is not a safe place to play.

Achieving High Organizational Momentum

Achieving an organizational level that is functioning with high momentum is an intentional, strategic, systematic process. You will not find a silver bullet to conquer this level but it is definitely obtainable. This book is dedicated to introducing the foundational core of healthcare environments to be able to achieve this level. Building high momentum or a core of excellence in healthcare begins with the colleagues first and foremost. Human capital is precisely that – CAPITAL.

There are no shortcuts, no hopscotch process for leading an organization to operating at a high momentum. Each step is important and the combination of all steps will compound and lead to creating an organization of high momentum. Applying the foundational principles in this book will be invaluable to help guide your organization to high momentum and great success.

Momentum Drainers

What can drain momentum in an organization? Review the list below and evaluate how often you observe these behaviors or attitudes within your organization:

* Distrust
* Confusion
* Negativity
* Selfishness
* Egocentric
* Verbal Abuse
* Financial Strain
* Control Seeking
* Poor Teamwork
* Poor Leadership
* Unresolved Conflict
* Vague Core Values
* Silo Mentality
* Lack of Vision and Mission
* Unprofessional Conduct
* Minimal Communication

Just one or a few of these behaviors or attitudes in an organization can create operational deficiencies and inefficiencies that are like a weight hanging over colleagues as they try to work. Positive high momentum is obtainable and should be the desire in order to have a highly functioning organization.

Momentum Builders

These are the behaviors and attitudes that leadership should seek to build high momentum within the cultural infrastructure of an organization. How frequently do you see them displayed in your organization?

- Trust
- Fairness
- Honesty
- Integrity
- Transparency
- Active Empathy
- Positive Attitudes
- Employee Engagement
- Reward and Recognition
- Employee Empowerment
- Team-focused Environment
- Clarity in Mission and Vision
- Valuing of Employee Strengths
- Effective Communication Pathways
- Competent Leadership at All Levels
- Competitive Compensation and Benefits
- Established Core Values
- Systems of Effective Workflow

Positive high momentum is easily detected and felt by colleagues and patients. Developing a culture of high momentum has to be a foundational priority for organizations.

Leaders Must Take the Lead.

I can hear the thoughts of some leaders as they read this. Are you thinking "I just do not understand all the hoopla about building momentum?"

Maybe you, like many, could say "there are too many internal and external pressures, challenges, and struggles just to stay afloat and to get through my 12-hour day." Or you feel that there is no time to work on momentum in your organization, deciding "I just need everyone to do their job and the organization will be fine."

I heard similar reactions from some staff when I took over the leadership of an organization that had a negative cash flow and held millions dollars of debt. Why would building momentum be important at this critical time when colleagues were losing their jobs, payroll not being met, and countless hours were needed to respond to angry vendors? It was an unspoken, collective question; asking "why be concerned about building momentum when we don't know if we are going to survive as an organization? Why add this little detail to the platter of problems?" But the fact remains that leaders cannot afford to delay creating specific strategies around building positive organizational energy or momentum. Particularly in dire circumstances, leadership must focus daily to cultivate positive momentum in their culture.

Turn Arounds

No organization is going to pull out of a nose dive without colleagues being an engaged part of the recovery. We need their energy to create the thrust to take us out of our valley of despair. Let's face it, the leadership cannot be the "end all" solution and many times they may not know the best solution to a problem. We need colleagues with different perspectives to deliver our best as healthcare organizations. Colleagues are our best secret weapon to the success for any organization. Not recognizing colleagues as the greatest asset of an organization pulls an organization down and creates a barrier to obtaining its true potential. The formula of poor leadership plus dissatisfied, disengaged colleagues yields trouble, often disaster. This does not have to be the case. Creating momentum is possible! Focusing on the principles portrayed in this book is a great way to begin.

My favorite saying as a healthcare leader is "sometimes I just need to get out of my colleague's way." I can do this confidently, because I trust my colleagues and know they will be the ones that will win each day in our organization. The core mass moving together builds excellence. Everyone wants to be successful in life. Why not allow colleagues to be successful in your organization? Having leadership who cast an engaging vision, and create a fertile work environment for personal and professional development will reverse negative momentum and move the organization toward achieving its highest possible level of success. Trust them and draw them into motion by involving and listening to them.

THE COLLEAGUE EXPERIENCE GENERATES MOMENTUM

So what does it take to have high momentum in an organization? The answer: momentum can only be achieved through the people of an organization, including each colleague regardless of title or position. Building momentum in an organization can be exciting, but must be intentional. The journey to high momentum is full of wonderful experiences for the leadership and employees. Savor the journey; it is very edifying to all.

Planning specific experiences by leadership to provide additional opportunities for colleague personal and professional growth within the organization brings momentum. The likelihood of momentum happening without well-planned strategies and execution would have similar odds to winning the lottery. It must be an intentional embraced process leadership and management.

There was a time in my leadership career that I felt that momentum could be achieved through what could be given to the colleague. Things such as higher salaries, raises, rewards, colleague lunches, family days, bonuses, flexible work schedules, college tuition program seemed to be the necessary steps. While each of these things are important to colleagues to show that they are appreciated and valued, I did not find these types of rewards to be very effective in building high momentum in the organization. While it made the organization attractive and more of an employer of choice, it could not take the place of what I refer to as authentic momentum. Authentic momentum comes from inside colleagues. It is not from external benefit. Momentum is an organic feature of an organization, grown from within colleagues.

I discovered that the level of positive momentum experienced in the organization was directly proportional to the colleague experience within the organization. One was dependent on the other. The more the colleagues from all areas of the organization were engaged on a personal and professional level, the greater the transformation of the organization toward success and the greater the momentum grew in the organization. An individual's personal momentum is as important as the organizations momentum. It begins with each individual first and then spills out into the organization.

This important discovery led me to create an environment that provided personal development of all colleagues – and I mean ALL colleagues. I am not referring to external continuing education, but internal personal and professional colleague development. The more colleagues are personally developed, engagement expands and the greater the momentum can be felt. Colleagues drive momentum. If you want your organization to continually improve and become successful, you must engage colleagues at a personal level. It takes investment, but the effort is worth it and the payoff is powerful for all stakeholders.

BEHAVIORS THAT DRIVE MOMENTUM

You can drive momentum by embedding these behaviors into your organization's culture:

+ Have total transparency of the financial situation.
+ Involve colleagues in the problem-solving process.
+ Focus on the strengths of the colleagues.
+ Cast a vision for "what could be."

* Continue to remind colleagues of this vision.
* Celebrate wins – both small and large.
* Work directly with the frontline staff to give them a place of importance and significance in the organization.
* Involve colleagues to assist in improving the work process, strategic planning and other initiatives
* Invite colleagues from all levels in the organization to teach organizational excellence workshops.

Frontline staff provides a driving force for maintaining positive momentum and are capable of constantly exceeding expectations. An organization's momentum can greatly impact the speed and direction of your organization. Colleagues are more likely to jump onto a fast moving train going in a defined direction than one that is stalling or limping along to a mysterious destination. Focusing on momentum is mandatory in leading an organization to excellence and beyond.

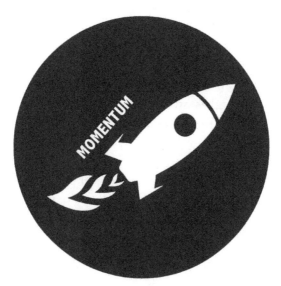

Figure 11

Our Momentum Symbol

The Corporate Transcendence™ Momentum Symbol[xlii] is a rocket in motion. Like most organizations, a rocket is a massively heavy, highly complex creation; getting one rocket to launch from ground level requires extensive expertise, large teams of well-trained individuals, and an immense amount of energy. People are the fuel cache in the organization; igniting them is the responsibility of leadership, and when they catch fire, the organization will be launched upward to another succeeding level.

Culture Transformation Action Steps:

Frontline Staff:

Regardless of your job title or the number of colleagues employed in your organization, representing a few hundred to thousands, colleagues directly contribute to momentum. Organizational momentum is sourced from the collective energy coming from colleagues. Your active engagement and empowerment in your work brings priceless energy. Personal energy has to be expressed, and it directly influences the quality and the flow intensity of momentum throughout the organization. Value and support positive momentum in your organization.

Managerial Leadership:

You have to first believe in your frontline colleagues. Give your front line the space to stretch their empowerment capacity. If you are struggling with this, dig back into the practice of valuing; recognize and affirm your staff and their strengths. Everyone has the internal desire to be more and do more. Give them space to grow and shine. Empower them effectively and they will be motivated to do more than what is expected.

Executive Leadership:

At the executive level you must always look at the momentum health of the organization. Exercise awareness of and address momentum busters like resource shortages or staffing issues. Recognize and reward the activities that build momentum. If you fail to recognize and reward the efforts that bring momentum, those efforts will fall off – and so will the momentum. Reward with things that matter to staff – like convenient parking and food or treats – can be an energy boost. Make sure to take care of your colleagues, helping them lift the weight of things they care for. If your people are bogged down long term, it will kill momentum. Continually focus on making it possible for colleagues to be successful in their work.

CHAPTER 12

Hardwiring: Success to Significance

• • •

Excellence is the gradual result of always striving to do better.

DEFINING SUCCESS

True success is multi-faceted; it is the optimization of the entire organization. Every area of an organization needs to be operating at optimal levels in order to lock into a successful state of existence. I discuss this process of locking in success as "hardwiring" your organization. This leads to replicability, and true transformation success that can lead to an even higher level of existence known as significance.

What does true success look like for the healthcare organization? The center core of success in healthcare relates back to the patient, the reason we exist. Success needs to be measured in how effective our care is to our patients. The many efforts, time and energy of the healthcare industry should be to create an organization that is able to function itself optimally in order to optimize the best possible healthcare outcomes for the patient.

Success in healthcare is not achieved in siloed activities. Corporate organizational success cannot be obtained by excellence achieved in a single area, department, function or operational process. The nature of healthcare functionality is too complex and interrelated to allow this. True success requires high levels of achievement in all functional areas, with performance that is consistent above average or outstanding.

A successful organization is like a healthy human physical body, with each organ and system complimenting each other and functioning at its best. In this analogy, all our human organs have purpose and contribute to having good health and livelihood. For example, the doctor doesn't save the life of a patient alone, there are hundreds and even thousands of supporting colleagues and people who are directly and indirectly involved to create the best care and a successful outcome for a patient. These individuals could be the direct care staff to the manufacturers of supplies and equipment or oversight entities that ensure safe and effective care of healthcare organizations, all coming together to provide best quality and safest care.

In a hardwired successful organization, repeated success equates to coming to the patient side with the highest possible colleague engagement and empowerment to support the best patient clinical outcomes possible. We move to success by breaking down the barriers and creating healthy culture in all areas: culture, quality, finance, and governance. Then hardwiring comes from continually improving, innovating and learning to benchmark against ourselves. Our purpose becomes to create transferrable, replicable tools and best practices. When we accomplish that, the hardwired success can produce significance.

THE PIPE DREAM

All leaders and colleagues working in healthcare desire to have a highly successful organization. The majority of all healthcare leaders work diligently, putting in many excessive hours to ensure the best for their patients is delivered. Upon arrival of new colleagues entering a new job position, there is a period of personal adaptation and socialization into the culture of the organization. The health of the culture they experience will be the direct result of what leadership has intentionally created, cultivated, nurtured and continue to develop within the organization. Leaders are the originators for cultural development and have the ultimate responsibility for maintaining a healthy culture for the organization. Leaders can chose to develop and foster a culture that is healthy and heals or a culture that is unhealthy and life threatening.

Leaders naturally desire a healthy thriving culture of excellence in their healthcare organization because it reflects their leadership ability. The challenge has been in how to accomplish this in our complex, demanding, complicated healthcare industry that seems to have thousands of simultaneous moving parts?

HEALTHCARE LANDSCAPE

Healthcare exist as a people industry composed of people taking care of people and in many instances at some of their most vulnerable and frightening experiences of their lives. This makes equipping healthcare colleagues and patients equally important to meet the high demands of successful healthcare. There is no such thing as business as usual, due to the uniqueness of working with numerous human characteristics in every part of its operations. Human beings with their innate emotions, strengths, weaknesses, changing life circumstances cannot be factored out of the healthcare success equation to achieve a desirable healthy cultural environment. Regardless of the fact that patients are who we serve, we cannot hopscotch over the caregivers and ignore their needs. When caregiver's needs are not addressed in a personal and professional manner, the healthcare environment is compromised and this drives potential serious outcomes for their patients. Just like a patient with a sickness, the healthcare environment and culture becomes sick and cannot function at its best.

Many healthcare organizations unequivocally have a deep cultural sickness. People who care for others have been found to be some of most caring people in the world. They deserve to work in a culture that allows them to be the most successful they can possibly be at doing what they enjoy and feel called to do. The following were results from a workshop on cultural transformation in which the 50 participants representing 10 different hospitals were asked "How would you describe healthcare in America?" Responses included: overwhelming, stressful, high anxiety, fear of job loss, complicated, complex, siloed, dysfunctional, competitive, hierarchical, chaotic, confusing, draining, and expensive. These are very disturbing answers and symptoms of a serious disease. Many of these colleagues have remained in this environment because of their love of caring for patients, but feel a level of dissatisfaction with their workplace. Their organizational culture is a major culprit to dissatisfaction.

The American healthcare environment is sick. It is seen in many ways as a culture that kills instead of a culture that heals. As many as 400,000 preventable annual patient deaths have been contributed to the care received in the healthcare environment. A root cause analysis reveals an organizational culture disorder as part of the problem.

Healthy culture transformation does not begin with the patient; it begins first and foremost with the caregivers. It is disappointing that an industry with such value to America and consisting of some of the most caring people on earth, is portrayed as one of the most dysfunctional industries that is overpriced, complex and complicated as well as splattered with documented preventable errors that do patients harm. It is truly time for transformation and the great news is transformation is achievable.

Healthcare has tested several business models that had been successful in many Wall Street companies. But an industry that is dealing with people suffering from life threatening illnesses, disease treatments and trauma, significant customization must be made. Completing a sales action as a customer in a retail store is not the same as discharging a patient from a hospital or registering in a patient to the emergency department or setting up tents to control Ebola in West Africa. Every industry has its own cultural needs to address in order to be successful, healthcare is no different.

We must cease hammering our square healthcare peg into a round business-as-usual hole. What is the multibillion dollar answer to saving the life of healthcare in America? The wonderful news is there is an answer and it does not need rocket science to achieve. It does take a different approach and innovation, thoughts and behaviors in daily operations. Every journey begins with a first step and this must be taken by focusing on creating a healthy culture within healthcare.

Blueprints for Success

The second natural question is how we create a culture that will deliver excellence that supports all areas of the organization. Factual there has never been a total comprehensive standardized blueprint for healthcare culture transformation, noticeable within healthcare history. There has been success in focusing on Patient Experience This question simply has not been a topic of much discussion. Now creating and sustaining a healthy cultural has become more like a mystery to be solved. Fragmentation or pieces of the transformation puzzle have been experimented with, but achieving organizational excellence has been many times short lived and the result of what seems to be happenstance and luck in many cases more than by intentional design.

The cultural health strategies of the past have not found themselves on the top ten priority leadership list and have been treated more like an add-on or a short term feel-good event for organizations, similar to taking a Tylenol for a headache. Focus on cultural health has consistently comprised of feel-good shooting stars or flavors of the months in attempts to improve or change a culture, with the objective of treating symptoms and not a disease. A standardized systemic universal methodology and curriculum of culture development for excellence has had limited discussion by collective leadership and now is emerging as a hot topic. Transformation of healthcare today becomes no longer optional but mandatory.

Many times, there is a tendency by leadership to focus the majority or 90 percent or more of their time on things that are uncontrollable. Governance or regulatory mandates come to healthcare providers mostly from outside sources. Medicare, Medicaid, commercial payers, the Patient Protection and Affordable Care Act, The Joint Commission, Health Resources and Services Administration (HRSA), state and local regulations are riddled with mandates for healthcare organizations. At the receiving end of these mandates it can feel like a large dump truck regularly backs up to the front door of the healthcare organization and dumps new and revised requirements for compliance without a survival guide or blueprint to model or demonstrate a proven pathway to be successful.

Healthcare organizations have many times become a victim to the Dump Truck Syndrome (DTS), instead of a victor. I am not saying that these regulatory requirements are not needed for safety and best care. However, these requirements have forced healthcare leaders to focus the majority of their time on the mandate and regulatory requirements and not on the healthcare culture that has to come first in order for the organization to be successful in meeting the requirements. Healthcare transformation of excellence is an inside out process. We must transform inside first to meet outside demands.

Non-controllable factors or additional external mandates will doubtfully decrease in the near future. Healthcare leaders are challenged to be able to cultivate an internal healthy culture that can survive the DTS. To accomplish this, the focus in healthcare leadership needs to be shifted, beginning with understanding the four essential cornerstones of excellence for leaders. These Four Cornerstones are culture, quality, finance, and governance.

CULTURE – PAC-MAN FOR SUCCESS

It cannot be overemphasized that the organization glue that holds organizational quality, finance and governance together begins with culture. Culture represents the healthcare worker factor within the organization that directly influences the health condition of the organization. Culture or organizational health has been neglected and healthcare culture needs a transformation. This first begins with culture and the necessary focuses that will begin to develop and create a culture of excellence. Culture is the protoplasm of the healthcare organizational cell in that it is the glue that will hold all organizational areas together. For that reason culture should be first priority in organizational transformation to excellence. For example, to transform an organization that is in looming bankruptcy, culture is priority and must come first. If the colleagues within the organization are not engaged the success of financial recovery will be limited. Culture eats everything in its path: operations, strategy, growth, and development. Cultivating and developing a culture of excellence begins with people and can make every day a success.

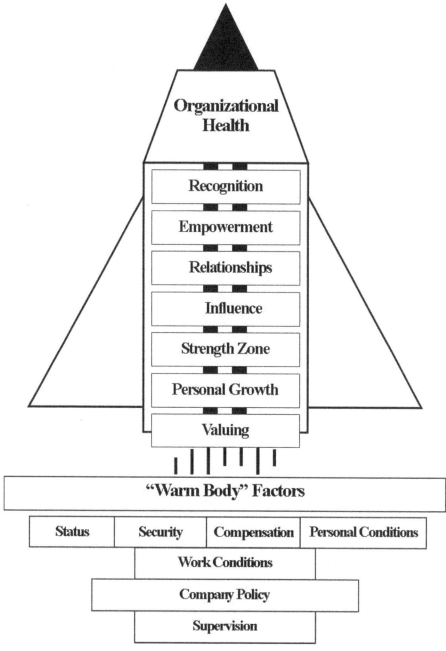

Figure 12: Corporate Transcendence Rocket

Hardwiring Components of Success

Healthcare leaders have many moving parts of an organization. Human Resources and Talent Management are vital components in healthcare organizations that healthcare leaders must monitor closely. There are many demands in regard to staffing, just to keep the doors open and operations running optimally. I refer to these as the warm body factors in my Corporate Transcendence™ Rocket illustrated.

The foundational block of the rocket is not an all-inclusive list, but serves to illustrate basic components considered and necessary to employ people. The what, when, how, or who factors are the expected items an organization must consider and or an applicant for employment would be looking for when considering a position with a company.

Status: What does the job description require?

Security: Is the organization financially stable?

Compensation: Are there competitive compensation and benefits?

Personal Conditions: Does this position fit my social factors, such as family obligations, travel time, work hours needs?

Work Conditions: Does it appear to be an aesthetically pleasing and friendly place to work and will I have the tools I need to perform my job?

Company policies: Do they align with legal employment standards and practices?

Supervision: Who will I report to and what will this relationship look like?

The components of this block are essential to attract people to consider working within healthcare of any organization. But the secret sauce of how an organization becomes an employer and provider of choice, and navigates an organization to success, excellence, transcendence and beyond is leadership investing into Corporate Transcendence™ Factors. These factors are applied universally to each colleague regardless of title, position, or job description. A curriculum that delivers greater influence, opportunity, and investment into each colleague is found through the intentional design of a corporate transcendent curriculum.

PERSONAL GROWTH

Healthcare professionals are seen many times as having it all together because of their highly esteemed profession and thought to have less personal needs since they are the designated caregivers. The fact is that due to performing in a complex people industry, they have a greater need to recharge and be exposed to opportunities of personal and professional development. Organizations that desire the best from their colleagues need to recognize that healthcare colleagues cannot give what they do not have. Serving in healthcare is demanding and can be extremely draining. Continuous attention to the healthcare colleague's well-being and development is essential for a culture of excellence.

Human beings innately need to expand, grow, and develop continuously. This is founded in natural, inborn tendencies as to whom we are as human beings. Each person can benefit from their own personal development experiences and time space for self-reflection. It is leadership's responsibility to make sure new colleagues and providers have multiple opportunities for personal development experiences within the work environment. When this does not occur, the employee will use their previous life experiences to filter their thoughts and behavior.

If we want to pull the best out of people, there has to be investment on the part of organizations. Give people what they naturally desire and they will give the organization what it needs to grow. Grow your colleagues and they will grow your organization in ways that you have never dreamed.

OPERATING IN STRENGTH ZONES

Identifying and valuing the strengths and assets that the healthcare colleagues bring to the organization pays off in great dividends for the organization. Strengths are like treasures that can be tapped into and utilized for the betterment of every aspect of the organization. Teams that recognize the strengths in their colleagues and how they complement others in team leadership find great success in problem solving and improving process. People living in their strength zones are more satisfied in their work and feel more fulfilled. Operating in their strength zone is edifying. Organizations need to invest in internal opportunities for colleagues to continually develop their strengths and build upon them.

INFLUENCE

People operating in their strength zone can develop greater positive influence among their colleagues Their strengths provides positive influence to their patients and will naturally seep into many areas of the organization. People need to feel safe to use their influence for the improvement of the responsibilities they are accountable for and for the organization as a whole entity. The power of positive influence among colleagues propels an organization in the desired direction to excellence, serving the colleague, patient and organization in the most rewarding way possible.

RELATIONSHIPS

Valuing all colleagues, personal development opportunities, working in our strength zones, and having a respectable voice of influence in our work environment will naturally build relationships and trust among all colleagues in an organization. Silos will break down. Continually developing stronger relationships with colleagues is a crucial part of sustaining a positive work environment. Relationships build trust and trust is needed to build high functioning teams. High functioning teams will develop greater excellence and best practices. The positive strength of a colleague's interrelationships in an organization will directly relate to its ongoing success.

EMPOWERMENT

To empower is to give up and share power. Empowerment stems from personal and professional development in healthcare. It creates positive synergy that propels the organization forward. By developing colleagues on a personal level, it is a natural step for them to take on more responsibility and accountability and utilize their new knowledge.

Empowerment creates shared power among colleagues and this is essential to having a highly functioning and reliability environment in healthcare. Empowerment is a true value in an organization and when properly initialized and developed it can take on a life of its own. Leaders who embrace this empowerment will observe a stimulating progressive environment that does not need micromanagement or leading. The best thing for leadership at this juncture of organizational development is to make sure they do not get in the way of progress and the continual steps to improvement and excellence that is propelled and owned by colleagues.

RECOGNITION

Rewarding by valuing and appreciating the commitment, dedication, hard work, strengths, and effort of colleagues has great payoffs. It does not have to or need to be always monetary in nature. There are many ways to recognize and hold valuable the great work of colleagues. Investing in colleagues personally and professionally within the organization grows the individual and the organization. No matter whom it is, being appreciated and demonstrating appreciation makes an impact on a person's self-worth. Positive reinforcement for work well done is essential. It supports accountability and continued growth in the organization.

TRANSCENDENCE

Remember valuing people, personal growth, operating within strength zones, possessing and allowing influence, relational strength among colleagues and leadership, empowerment among colleagues, recognition and appreciation for colleagues' hard work and efforts will create repeated success, excellence, and significance for organizations in healthcare and in any other industry.

INTENTIONAL SUCCESS

Successful transformation of an organization to excellence will come by utilizing strategic systemic sustainable solutions. Organizations do not simply chance upon excellence. When there is not a deliberate intentional systemic approach to develop a culture of excellence, it will be a culture of competing cultures. In other words, what the employee brings to the organization from their personal and professional experiences will define the culture of the organization. If you take an organization with 5,000 employees, the subcultures are compounded based on personal and professional experiences of the employees in all walks of their lives. The cultures will be a smorgasbord of thoughts, values, beliefs, behaviors, expectations, and various culture behaviors will swirl throughout the organization daily. Each person will have their own unique perception of the organization and how they would describe its operations and norms.

Colleagues with different perception, and thus a different reality, lead to competing realities in the workplace. Leaders cannot verbalize the reality of their organization they desire to have without modeling and putting action to their words through experiences and observations the colleague has the opportunity to experience.

For example, an employed physician experiences disconnect between the hospital leadership and the medical staff. There is a poor relationship and the two parties develop distrust. Throwing each party under the bus may have been a common occurrence. This infects other and the medical staff begins to feel as an entity that the leadership only cares about the bottom line, and leadership feels that the medical staff just wants all the expensive and latest medical toys to do their job without thought to the financial impact to the hospital. This type of silo disconnect atmosphere in healthcare has in many occasion existed. For examples, there can be functioning disconnection issues between departments, like surgery and laboratory, medical imaging and cardiopulmonary or environmental services and housekeeping. Walls of silos can exist in healthcare organization anywhere.

Now, consider a medical doctor graduating from medical school enters a different healthcare culture that shares all financial, culture, quality, and governance information with the medical staff and engages the medical staff into conversations and discussions around these topics. The organization appears to value and respect all people and their opinions from any position of the organizations. Everyone has an opportunity to speak and be listened to. The new staff members had never experienced this before. This vastly differs from the culture that the new medical provider spent their years of residency in. Naturally, they would be skeptical and distrusting of this new culture, until the staff member experiences the new culture at many levels of consciousness.

CULTURAL TRANSFORMATION TAKES TIME

Transforming culture time factor is dependent on how deep the diseased culture is embedded in the organization. It relies on how internal and external factors are impacting an organization. If an organization is in severe financial distress that is a sure sign that transformation must take place, for example at a robust change rate. If an organization is not in financial distress and is financially stable, but for example is experiencing employee turnover due to low morale, then the pace of transformation can be expedited in a more gradual pace in the organization, but definitely needs immediate attention. Gradual does not mean a lackadaisical approach. Cultural momentum is dependent on building positive energy and can easily decline if not hardwired strategically in the organization.

Transform Your Culture

The good news is that cultural transformation from a sick culture to a culture that heals is highly achievable for any healthcare organization regardless of its size. It does require certain nonnegotiable principles to exist. It is up to leadership and governance to decide if they desire their organization to be a poor, average or mediocre, above average, excellent or a transcendent organization. These decisions will land squarely on the shoulders of the leadership of the organization. Sorry, no excuses accepted.

This requires among all stakeholders levels, new thought innovation and processing by healthcare leaders. It will require a peeling away of traditional hierarchical thinking and leading that needs to be removed. Partnering and team leadership is essential for success within and outside our healthcare industry walls. Leaders in healthcare must be innovated in developing excellence as a norm to take our American healthcare system from being a healthcare system in the world that spends the most money on healthcare and have some of the worst patient health outcomes, to being the best healthcare leader in the world. The solutions or truth lay within the walls of healthcare leaders and colleagues minds.

As healthcare colleagues, will we take the challenge to heal our healthcare culture in order to meet the challenges of our present healthcare environment or continue to repeat the past, by treating the symptoms of our unhealthy culture? Having an industry with human lives are at stake, filled with healthcare colleagues with amazing compassion and valuable strengths and talents, there is no reason why American healthcare culture cannot experience excellence of a transcendent nature now and into the future.

There are 18 million healthcare workers in America while the expected need is 5.6 million more by the year 2020. As healthcare leaders, and all the people who have a stake in the system, it is time to reframe our healthcare entities with a systematic approach to creating a culture that HEALS.

Successes or wins are the first milestone marker on the way to hardwiring an organization of excellence. The leg on the journey is filled with not only continuous improvements in culture, quality, finance, and governance, but with the spirit of enlightenment and innovation. A higher level of self-reflecting, sensitivity to subtle details for refining and a proactive consciousness and the capacity to flex, adjust and change operations should be accepted and expected among colleagues. Working as interdisciplinary team, valuing each person's contribution, expertise and thought process is the normal culture. The organization is able to replicate their successes in all departments through solid workflow processes. The number of best practices continually grows and expands. Cutting edge evidence-based medicine and care is genuinely developed and embraced.

MOVING BEYOND SUCCESS TO SIGNIFICANCE

This highly successful replicability culture is the linchpin for hardwiring an organization that exists within a culture of ongoing and expectant success, to one of significance. Significance is the summit peak of a healthy organization. Success is a more quantifiable measure of an action or event. It is tangible and more easily identifiable. Success can many times be more siloed and measured in growth, money, quantity, outcomes, and the accumulation of things. Success in healthcare will require a cross-functional team working together in all areas, frontline engagement and fertile environment to foster engagement, empowerment and innovation within all colleagues regardless of title or position. Success will be the outcomes and the cultural norm mindset and anything different feels off balance or weird. Success is the normal expectation of all colleagues. Constant energy expedited by all colleagues to look for improvements in all areas of work, understanding that success and excellence is a journey and not a destination. The culture propels itself to seek continuous excellence as a high reliability organization.

Becoming an organization of significance means the organizations respiration and pulse exemplifies the organization's core values. The mindset of proactive continuous improvement in all areas of the organization becomes transferable and replicable. This is what propels an organization to its own self-awareness and its significance.

From this point significance as an organization is achieved through reliability, hardwiring and the evergreen process, for a culture of sustainable success. Achieving significance results from the ongoing accomplishment of success, but is of a greater value. Significance has a long life or leaves a legacy of excellence. It invests in ways that are long lasting for patient's health and quality of life. It invests in the personal and professional development of those that provide care. It builds a succession of highly competent leaders and healthcare workers that has DNA of success, significance and transcendence, seeking extraordinary results in all they do to elevate the whole being of their fellow man.

REPLICATING SUCCESS

Just because you have success does not mean you have arrived! Hardwiring is not about arriving at an appointed destination. In order to hardwire, we continuously benchmark our performance, care provided and patient clinical outcome against our history in order to continuously innovate and improve. An organization at this level is never satisfied or plateauing. The organization consistently invests in the patient, one another, and the community. At this specific time an organization is hardwired for not only success but significance. Hardwiring an organization recognizes that it requires continual innovation and investment in the patients, colleagues, community – and getting good at generating replicable success. You must replicate success in order to achieve significance.

The significance level is not always about building another hospital or clinic. It is about making a real difference in the patient's lives – and our colleague's lives. If we really help people manage their health better, and live a longer life – that is so much greater than measuring our success in dollars and cents. Significance is felt when we are making a difference in people's lives and the world.

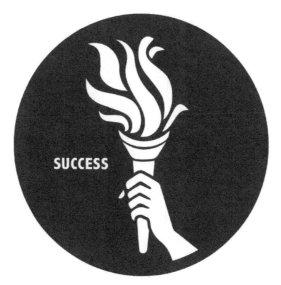

Figure 13

Our Success Symbol

The Corporate Transcendence™ Success Symbol[xliv] is a continuously flaming torch. Success is not an event. It is the ongoing replicability of successful processes composed of the greatest values being brought forward by every direct and indirect caregiver set of hands. The flaming torch Success Symbol recognizes an organization and the numerous daily actionable steps that will result in the highest quality level of care. The torch flame burns continuously regardless of and internal or external influencing factors, or hour of the day in the healthcare environment. The Success Flame represents a continual hardwiring of multiple best practices composed of evidence-based care that is always improving and making a sound progressive difference in the healthcare delivery of care environment. Just like in the Olympics where people train and develop to benchmark against others, as well as their last best achievable record of excellence, the flaming torch symbol is a reminder that there is always room for improvement and progress to be made in caring for people's health. This symbol's purpose is to make sure this truth is not forgotten or extinguished.

Pamela M. Tripp

Culture Transformation Action Steps:

Frontline Staff:
Hardwiring success and excellence in the organization is the product of collective thinking. The organizational mind reflects what it sees modeled. It must be favorable toward continued learning opportunities to stretch for success. This requires a personal intentional strategy. Frontline staff should seize opportunities to engage in their work setting and continually expand their thinking. The greatest source of ideas, innovation, and problem-solving is frontline healthcare staff. Strive to become and help colleagues to be a catalyst for success and ultimate significance. Your legacy will shine through.

Managerial Leadership:
Valuing all colleagues through relationship leadership is essential to being effective. A single manager cannot win the day, but engaging your team and letting their strengths be utilized and appreciated will build an awesome team of healthcare colleagues that will make a difference daily for safe and effective care. Managers orchestrate the team building processes. Never settle for status quo in yourself or others. Be an innovator of excellence and a mentor of quality for your team's success.

Executive Leadership:
The weight of success and excellence is shouldered upon executive leadership. Embrace an intentional strategic vision for cultural transformation that will remain steadfast as an essential ongoing priority. Leadership is expected to be openly portrayed in an organization as the ultimate mentor for creating an accountability environment of excellence. Valuing all colleagues first and using their strengths as an engaging and empowering bedrock of success will yield excellence, and ultimately organizational significance that impacts people in your community, state, nation and beyond.

Conclusion

• • •

To obtain a vision, it is said to begin with the arrival point in mind. Bringing this book to its end is not the completion of a vision, but the foundation of it. This book represents a greater effort on my behalf to share with as many people as possible the truths learned in my journey to support healthcare culture transformation to excellence and transcendence. This full vision will be achieved when the reality of America's healthcare industry is ranked the best in the world.

All visions have beginning steps or stages and require a strong and enduring foundation. The principles shared in this book are the fertile soil for the roots from the Trees of Transcendence (culture, quality, finance, and governance) to grow in. I share the importance of these trees of strength in my Corporate Transcendence™ Transformation Curriculum program. From a tree roots typically grow deep and spread out in the ground as a tree matures. Roots are not normally seen, but their role is unmistakable. They are the conduits through which the nourishments from nutrients and water are feed to the tree to maintain life. The roots support the tree trunk, limbs and branches, just like the foundational principles of this book supports healthcare transformation.

My vision comes from my burning passion and desire to continue serving organizations to support their journey of transformation to excellence and beyond to transcendence.

I close with these words of wisdom from an unknown author, by challenging the reader to become the Eagle of Excellence that you and your colleagues were born to become:

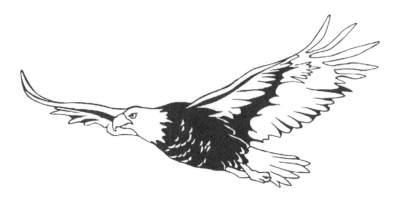

"What you settle for stays with you. Why settle for average when you can be phenomenal? Why live in a chicken coup when you can soar like an eagle? You are the gatekeeper of your destiny. Shut the door to ordinary and open your life to extraordinary."

Corporate Transcendence
Work Culture Survey

Please evaluate each statement using the following ranking system, and check the corresponding box to give your evaluation.   Use the sum to evaluate your culture for opportunities for growth.

1 - Strongly Disagree   2 - Disagree   3 - Neither Agree nor Disagree   4 - Agree   5 - Strongly Agree   Score

1 2 3 4 5

Statement	Score
This organization is seen as an employer of choice.	____
My employees with leadership titles inspire others to lead.	____
My employees with leadership titles engage direct reports in team leadership.	____
Employees are encouraged to view themselves as leaders in their area of responsibility.	____
Employees are encouraged to question the status quo without fear, intimidation, or retaliation.	____
Employees are given opportunities to grow personally and professionally in my organization.	____
Internal promotions are considered and encouraged in my organization.	____
Employees understand the mission and vision of the organization.	____
Employees appear to understand their personal strengths and use them effectively in daily operations.	____
Employees are highly motivated to contribute their best in the work place.	____
Employees believe excellence in areas of quality, finance, culture, governance is obtainable.	____
Employees feel valued and cared for in this organization.	____
Leaders model and coach employees for excellence at all levels of the organization.	____
We have high-functioning interdisciplinary teams.	____
In our environment we have open communication, transparency, and room to grow through mistakes.	____
All levels of leadership seem themselves as role models and mentors to their employees.	____
This organization provides resources to guide leaders and employees to significantly improve.	____
Leadership seems confident and strongly committed to the *excellence journey* for this organization.	____
Young and struggling leaders are coached and feel encouraged.	____
Employees have the tools and resources to improve their work environment.	____
Employees feel hope, empowerment, and personal significance from being associated with the company.	____
Employees' strengths are tapped and utilized to support a work culture of excellence.	____
This organization's culture values individual workers as a fellow human being regardless of position or title.	____
This organization provides a clear curriculum for employees to achieve excellence.	____
Frontline employees play a role in creating a culture of excellence.	____
All levels of the organization function in unity, with empowered teams for independent problem solving.	____
Leaders and employees leave work energized, eagerly anticipating the next workday.	____
Leaders and employees speak highly of their job and recommend their organization as a great place to work.	____
My organization produces and provides world class products and services.	____

Total for Your Score ____

Score of 0-79	0-79 Your organization has an urgent need for culture transformation.
Score of 80-114	80-114 Your organization has the opportunity for improvement in multiple areas.
Score of 115-136	115-136 Your organization is positioning itself for Excellence.
Score of 137-145	137-145 Your organization is positioned for sustainable excellence.

Illustrations

• • •

Learn More

• • •

Learn More about Corporate Transcendence™

To learn more about the Corporate Transcendence™ culture transformation curriculum, visit www.CorporateTranscendence.com. If you are interested in transforming your healthcare organization, or would like to invite Pamela M. Tripp to speak to your convention or organization, visit the Corporate Transcendence™ website to contact her team.

Further Writing by Pamela M. Tripp

For free resources and to be notified of Pamela's upcoming books, visit her author website, www.PamelaTripp.com. There you will be able to read her articles and keep up with her activities. For access to exclusive free culture assessment and leadership support resources, register for her email list. Subscribers receive exclusive content that can help executive and frontline healthcare leaders begin turning the tide.

About the Author

• • •

Pamela M. Tripp, MEd, MSOM

Pamela Tripp is driven by her life's passion for building the best healthcare system in America and the world. Her starting place begins with organizational health in making sure our healthcare industry develops a culture that heals instead of a culture that kills. Pamela has garnered extensive experience as a healthcare educator, thought leader, senior executive, and turnaround CEO. Pamela has spent the last 20 years perfecting and testing a transformational curriculum to deliver sustainable healthcare excellence in culture, quality, finance, and governance.

As Pamela's break out book *The Culture Cure* introduces 9 foundational principles to lay the groundwork for building an organization of transcendence. Believing that true healthcare transformation begins from the inside out, Pamela shares her conclusion that innovation for an excellent healthcare system comes from the ones who know it the best – healthcare leaders and colleagues.

As CEO of CommWell Health, Pamela led this large healthcare system from bankruptcy to achieve the North Carolina Governor's Malcolm Baldrige First Milestone award in 6 short years. Pamela was the first recipient of the Founders President award from Custom Learning of Canada for Exemplary Leadership in Service Excellence, and her organization has received more than 36 national service excellence awards for best practices, patient satisfaction, and healthcare innovation. Pamela serves on the North Carolina Community Health Center Board and the national

Health Choice Network board representing 27 community health centers nationwide. She is a member of the American College of Healthcare Executives and earned VIP status with the National Association of Professional Women. Pamela is the founder of the Johnston Community College "Women in Leadership" endowment.

Pamela is certified by leadership expert John C. Maxwell with Mentorship status bringing extensive training and experience in developing the leadership within her organization and everyone she touches. Learn more about Pamela at www.PamelaTripp.com and follow her on social media for ongoing insights and encouragement from the frontlines of healthcare transformation in the United States of America.

References

• • •

1   Common Wealth Fund. US Health System Ranks Last Among Eleven Countries on Measures of Access, Equity, Quality, Efficiency, and Healthy Lives. http://www.commonwealthfund. org/publications/press-releases/2014/jun/us-health-system-ranks-last. Accessed February 12, 2016.

2   The Center for Appreciative Inquiry. Home Page. http://www.centerforappreciativeinquiry.net. Accessed July 6, 2016.

4   The Corporate Transcendence™ Vision Symbol is property of Corporate Transcendence™ and may not be used or reproduced without express permission.

5   Common Wealth Fund. US Health System Ranks Last Among Eleven Countries on Measures of Access, Equity, Quality, Efficiency, and Healthy Lives. http://www.commonwealthfund. org/publications/press-releases/2014/jun/us-health-system-ranks-last. Accessed February 12, 2016.

6   The Joint Commission. http://www.jointcomission.org. Accessed July 6, 2016.

7   CommWell Health. http://www.commwellhealth.org/. Accessed July 6, 2016.

8   Lean Six Sigma. Wikimedia Foundation; June 22, 2016. https://en.wikipedia.org/wiki/lean_six_sigma. Accessed July 6, 2016.

9   NIST. Baldrige Performance Excellence Program. http://nist.gov/baldrige. Accessed July 6, 2016.

10 Corporate Memory Solutions. http://corporatememorysolutions.com. Accessed July 6, 2016.

11 Hospital Consumer Assessment of Healthcare Providers and Systems. http://hcahpsonline.org. Accessed July 6, 2016.

12 HHS.gov U.S. Department of Health & Human Services. http://hhs.gov. Accessed July 6, 2016.

13 Accountable Care Organizations (ACO). Centers for Medicare & Medicaid Services. https://www.cms.gov/aco/. Accessed July 6, 2016.

About the National Quality Strategy (NQS). Agency for Healthcare Research and Quality. http://www.ahrq.gov/workingforquality/about.htm#aims. Accessed July 6, 2016.

15 Berwick DM, Nolan TW, Whittington J. The Triple Aim: Care, Health, and Cost. http://content.healthaffairs.org/content/27/3/759.long. Accessed February 12, 2016.

16 Centers for Medicare & Medicaid Services. cms.gov. Accessed July 6, 2016.

17 World Bank Group. World Development Indicators. http://apps.who.int/nha/database/Select/Indicators/en. February 12, 2016.

19   The Corporate Transcendence™ Leadership Symbol is property of Corporate Transcendence™ and may not be used or reproduced without express permission.

20   Keller S, Price C. Organizational health: The ultimate competitive advantage. http://www.mckinsey.com/insights/organization/organizational_health_the_ultimate_competitive_advantage. Accessed February 12, 2016.

21   LaBier. The New Resilience. Are You Suffering From Empathy Deficit Disorder? https://www.psychologytoday.com/blog/the-new-resilience/201004/are-you-suffering-empathy-deficit-disorder. Accessed February 16, 2016.

22   Gordon M. Roots of Empathy: Who we are. http://www.rootsofempathy.org/en/who-we-are.html. Accessed February 16, 2016.

23   Harvard Graduate School of Education. The Making Caring Common Project. http://sites.gse.harvard.edu/making-caring-common/about. Accessed February 12, 2016.

24   Weissbourd R, Jones S. How Parents Can Cultivate Empathy in Children. http://sites.gse.harvard.edu/sites/default/files/making-caring-common/files/empathy.pdf. Accessed February 12, 2016.

26   The Corporate Transcendence™ Empathy Symbol is property of Corporate Transcendence™ and may not be used or reproduced without express permission.

28   The Corporate Transcendence™ Ownership Symbol is property of Corporate Transcendence™ and may not be used or reproduced without express permission.

29 Sharkey P, Elwert F. THE LEGACY OF DISADVANTAGE: MULTIGENERATIONAL NEIGHBORHOOD EFFECTS ON COGNITIVE ABILITY. American Journal of Sociology. 2011;116(6). http://www.ncbi.nlm.nih.gov/pmc/articles/PMC3286027/. Accessed July 8, 2016.

30 Conwell RH. Acres of Diamonds. http://www.temple.edu/about/history/acres-diamonds. Accessed February 12, 2016.

32 The Corporate Transcendence™ Personal Strengths Symbol is property of Corporate Transcendence™ and may not be used or reproduced without express permission.

34 Maslow AH. A Theory of Human Motivation. Psychological Review. 1943;50:370-396.

36 The Corporate Transcendence™ Equipping Symbol is property of Corporate Transcendence™ and may not be used or reproduced without express permission.

38 The Corporate Transcendence™ Empowerment Symbol is property of Corporate Transcendence™ and may not be used or reproduced without express permission.

39 Positivity. Positivity Ratio. https://www.positivityratio.com/. Accessed July 8, 2016.

40 Losada M, Heaphy E. The role of Positivity and Connectivity in the performance of business teams: A Nonlinear dynamics model. American Behavioral Scientist. 2004;47(6):740–765. doi:10.1177/0002764203260208.

42 The Corporate Transcendence™ Momentum Symbol is property of Corporate Transcendence™ and may not be used or reproduced without express permission.

44 The Corporate Transcendence™ Success Symbol is property of Corporate Transcendence™ and may not be used or reproduced without express permission.